MW00342885

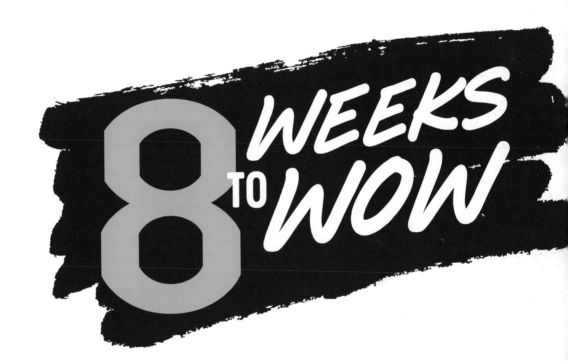

8 WEEKS TO WOW

EMILIE BRABON-HAMES & CHIEF BRABON

MURDOCH BOOKS

SYDNEY · LONDON

WHO WILL YOU BE 8 WEEKS FROM NOW?

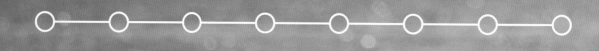

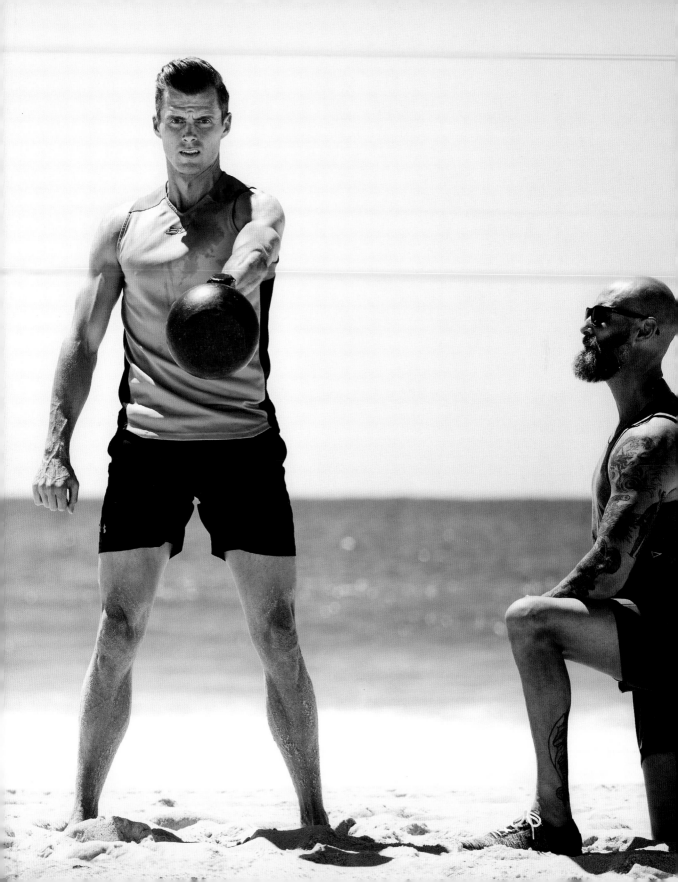

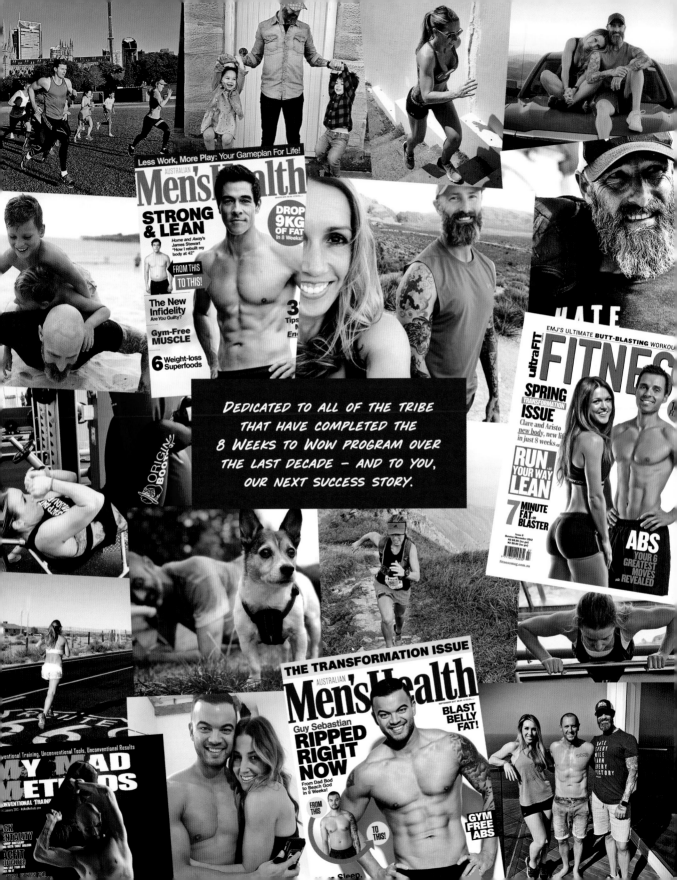

DEDICATED TO ALL OF THE TRIBE
THAT HAVE COMPLETED THE
8 WEEKS TO WOW PROGRAM OVER
THE LAST DECADE — AND TO YOU,
OUR NEXT SUCCESS STORY.

WELCOME	06
GUY'S STORY	16
JULES'S STORY	18

THE LIST 20

THE LIST AT A GLANCE	26

THE DARC WORKOUTS 30

WEEKS 1–2	34
WEEKS 3–4	42
WEEKS 5–6	50
WEEKS 7–8	58

THE WEEKS 66

WEEK 1	68
CHRISTINA'S STORY	70
WEEK 2	80
ANDY'S STORY	82
WEEK 3	88
RICHARD & REBECCA'S STORY	90

WEEK 4	96
SHARLEEN'S STORY	98
WEEK 5	104
PATRICK'S STORY	106
WEEK 6	112
CONNIE'S STORY	114
WEEK 7	118
DUSTIN'S STORY	120
WEEK 8	126
ROSIE'S STORY	128

THE RECIPES 132

WEEK 1	134
WEEK 2	144
WEEK 3	158
WEEK 4	170
WEEK 5	180
WEEK 6	188
WEEK 7	196
WEEK 8	206

YOU MADE IT!	214
INDEX	218
THANKS, TRIBE!	223

WELCOME TO YOUR VERY OWN 8-WEEK TRANSFORMATION!

Over the past 10 years, the team behind the 8 Weeks to Wow (8WTW) program that Chief and I created have produced jaw-dropping results – beyond anything the health and fitness industry has ever seen.

Initially, this eating plan came about when Chief and I were hired to turn 13 fit, but not toned, individuals into Lycra-clad warriors in only 6 weeks for the 2008 hit television series *Gladiators*. Many of the fitness professionals who were approached claimed that it would be simply impossible to achieve the desired results in 6 weeks, but we took up the challenge. The objectives were clear: strip away excess fat, increase the athletes' strength, speed and endurance, and most importantly (as Lycra is an unforgiving fabric) give them great muscle tone. The men needed to look powerful and awe-inspiring, while the women had to have that rare balance of femininity and athleticism. Despite our limitations, the outcome was nothing less than amazing.

After the success of those transformations, we were asked by our Original Bootcamp and personal training clients if they could use the same eating plan, in addition to following our workout routines. Of course, the 6-week plan needed to be adjusted to suit everyday people with families, so our plan evolved into the 8 Weeks to Wow program. Once we launched the first mainstream 8WTW program, the word spread fast. When people realised the kind of results that were possible in a relatively short amount of time, they were thrilled. And, unlike other diets, they found that the results stuck and were pleasantly easy to maintain.

Our transformations have featured on the covers of major magazines and in scores of media articles. They've been seen by international visitors, who have read about our program and wanted to take part themselves. Year round, there are people from all over the world participating in 8WTW – people from Australia, France, the UK and all over America. This group includes workers on deep-sea oil rigs, as well as soldiers in Afghanistan, families in Hong Kong and individuals living in the most rural parts of Australia. These people all have one thing in common: they are committed to change.

Since 2008, when we launched 8WTW to a broader audience, our program has had literally thousands of success stories – people whose lives have been transformed immeasurably. We have heard so many different stories, from people dropping a clothing

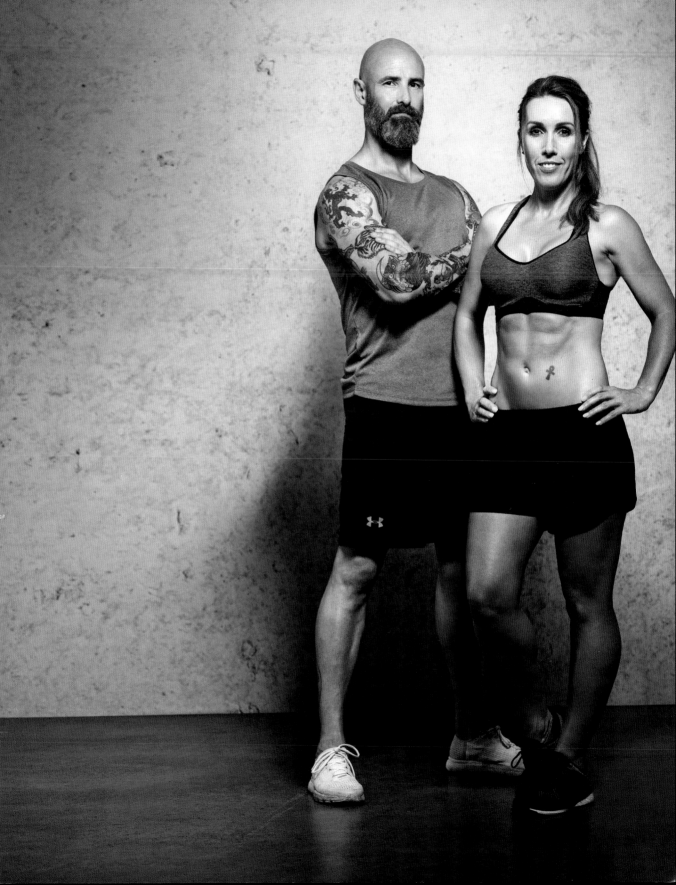

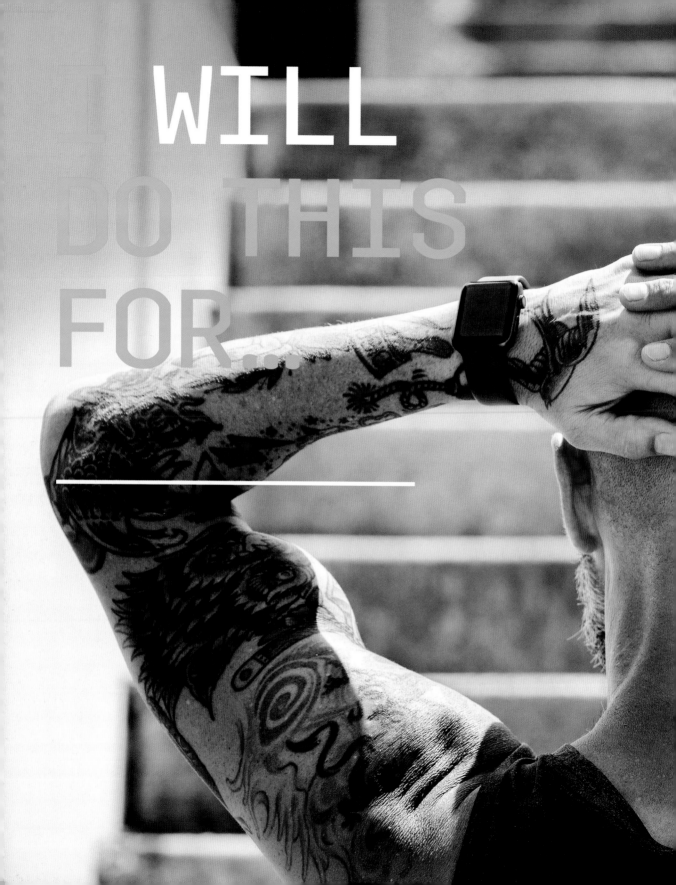

I WILL

DO THIS

FOR...

_____

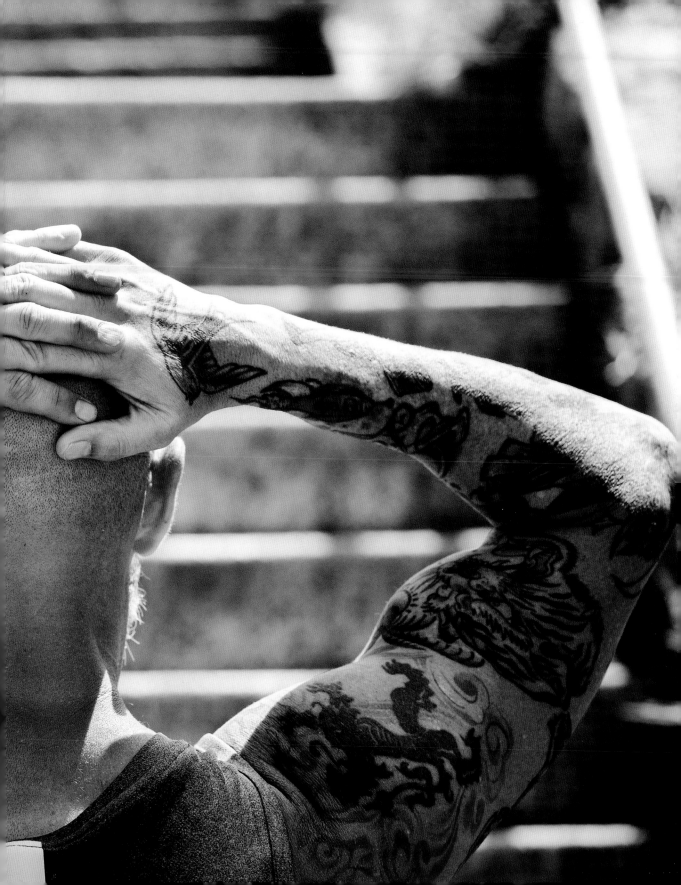

size or ten, becoming fitness models, feeling so much happier in themselves and, most importantly, people unshackling themselves from the myriad health issues that are associated with being overweight, including Type 2 diabetes, high blood pressure and fertility complications. Participants in our program have entered physique competitions, run marathons, competed in iron man challenges and triathlons. Some have even returned to professional sports.

The 8WTW program is an 8-week commitment to change – it involves getting used to new ideas, new workouts and new flavours. The best part is that it's achievable for anyone ready to make that commitment to themselves. Whether you have a family or you keep crazy working hours and have limited time for training, 8WTW can fit into your busy schedule. We know this because we've seen people do it time and time again.

YOU ARE WHAT YOU EAT

A huge part of the 8WTW plan is, of course, the food that you fuel your body with. Our eating plan has evolved from a training program for elite athletes to a program for everyday people and everyday athletes who want to get fit – fast.

The aim of 8WTW is to reboot your mindset and your body so that it can best use the foods you are eating. We call it a 'metabolic optimisation' eating plan. Basically, it's a high-protein, low-fat and super-low-carb plan that's designed to reset your body's resting metabolic rate. And that means burning more fat, all the time.

We have developed the 8WTW program in collaboration with chefs, dietitians, nutritionists, GPs and physiologists, so you can be assured of its effectiveness and the positive changes it will have on your body and mind. But everyone's situation is unique, so if you do have any existing health issues, it goes without saying that you need to consult your doctor before you start, to make sure the program fits in with your treatment plan.

The foundation of our food plan is something called 'The List', and it is (you've guessed it) a master list of the foods you should be eating at different points in this program. Don't panic if your favourite thing to eat isn't on our list. Remember, this is ONLY 8 weeks of your life – it's not forever. The ingredients on The List are there for a reason: these are the foods we've found most effective for this plan. Who knows – you may even discover a few new favourites!

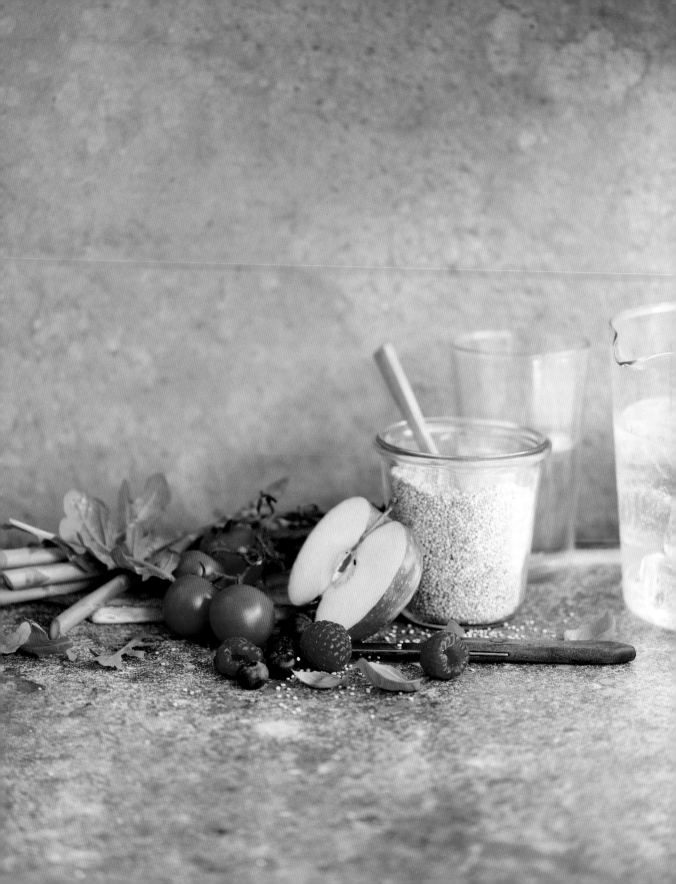

To ensure that your time on the 8WTW program is not just rewarding but also pleasurable, we've chosen the most delicious and easy recipes from our online plan. They're so good that you won't feel as though you're missing out . Being able to enjoy satisfying food will help you achieve better results. If there are things on The List that you don't like, simply work around them. And as for all those foods you love, like fruit, rice, pasta and nuts, you'll gradually reintroduce them into your diet at the right time. It will work; it just takes some commitment. And, unlike other diets and fads that you may have tried, you won't regain the weight you lose, as long as you don't go back to your old habits.

WHAT SETS 8 WEEKS TO WOW APART?

By far the most common question we get here at 8WTW HQ is this: What makes the 8WTW program different from all the other programs out there?

The answer is simple: There are hundreds of scientific ways to lose weight and burn body fat; some are fast, some are slow, some are easy and some are hard. The one thing that many of these programs don't do is teach your body how to use the food you're eating for its optimum purpose. The aim of the 8WTW program is to 'reboot' your metabolism so it learns to use fat as a primary source of fuel on a day-to-day basis, in a process called ketosis. Many people find it hard to stick to a ketogenic diet because we're all quite addicted to our carbs. So at 8WTW, we take the carbs away for just a few weeks, giving your metabolism a nice little 'keto kickstart', before slowly introducing them back into your diet.

Over the years, portion sizes in the Western world have become much bigger than our stomach size. We are eating way too many carbs in the wrong way, but we're going to help you fix that. Let's call it a metabolic reboot.

We kickstart this reboot by removing certain food groups entirely, and by ensuring you are hydrated enough for your body to function properly. And we provide you with all the necessary information to ensure you're living in a much more carb-conscious way by the time this program is over. We want you to understand and respect portion sizes, recognise the different food groups and also understand the necessity of eating the right foods at the right time. That's how you're going to transform for life.

The program works in the long term for every body shape, age and size – male or female, time poor or time rich. And it isn't just for people who are overweight; it's been designed to shape and tone your body into a physique that most people only dream of. The benefits of this change are endless, from simple things like feeling amazing, to being able to chase your kids around the yard without running out of breath, to one of the most important things: having peace of mind that you have a healthy body and mind .

There are really only three things you need to master to make the 8WTW program work for you:

[1] Drink 2 litres (70 fl oz/8 cups) of water each day
[2] Exercise 5–6 days a week
[3] Follow the eating plan by sticking to The List of allowed foods

Follow these few simple rules, and you'll have the body you want, for as long as you want. Change your mindset, and change your life!

Since the inception of the original version that the *Gladiator* contestants took part in, many of our successful and incredibly amazing-looking participants have graced the covers of magazines, advertisements and newspapers. Now we want YOU. It's your turn to have the body, mindset and way of life that you've always wanted. Exert just a little bit of willpower, and that dream is only 8 weeks away.

WELCOME TO THE TRIBE.

Em & Chief Brabon

ROLE

MODELS

~~NOT~~

~~INSTA~~

~~MODELS~~

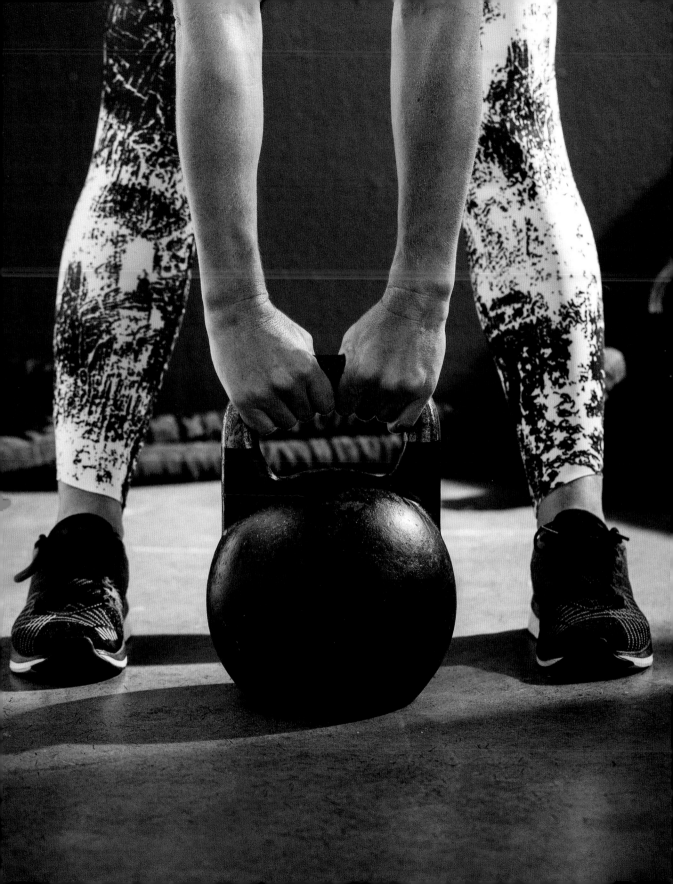

TRANSFORMATION STORIES
GUY'S STORY

Name: Guy Sebastian

Age: 36

Occupation: Singer/Songwriter

When did you complete the 8WTW program? Mid 2017

What motivated you to undertake this program?
At first, I took on the program to finally get to that next level of fitness. For years I'd tried, but I just couldn't break through. Another motivation was constant chronic pain. I grew up playing AFL and cricket, and had injured my back and hip. The pain was getting quite severe and I'd been told three times to have surgery. After research, I decided to try and fix the problems that caused these injuries to get worse. I needed to strengthen my core and other muscles I didn't know existed. As far as pain management, the results have been mind-blowing.

What goals did you set for yourself?
Well, those goals kind of got set for me – turned out my manager at the time was in talks with *Men's Health*. Doing a cover for them was all the motivation I needed! I was never a 'get your shirt off in public' bloke so it was extremely daunting. My goals were to not give up and to get off my pain medication.

Did you meet those goals?
Absolutely. I actually shocked myself. I hadn't seen my abs since I was young – before most of my time was spent sitting in studios and moving the computer mouse around writing songs!

Which aspect of the program did you find the most challenging?
The diet part was tough. I wasn't a terrible eater, but I realised that the little things count. Sugars in coffees, eating late at night and eating too much were all blocking my progress. The first 5 weeks were seriously tough! But then I got to this point where I just didn't need bad food anymore. I'm still at that point. I have power over those desires and treat myself in a controlled manner. I should also add that my injuries were killing me for those first 5 weeks. I nearly gave up several times, it was bloody hard work but then something clicked, and for the first time in years the pain stopped – it was like magic.

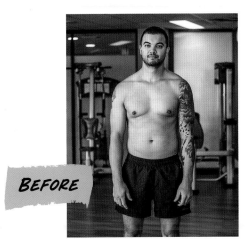

BEFORE

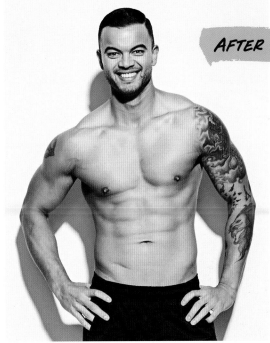

AFTER

Which week was the hardest for you? Why?

Any of those first 4-5 weeks because of the food change and pain. After that it was all focus – I got addicted to that clear feeling in my head and that determination carried through my day.

Favourite exercise from the workouts?

Favourite is a strange word to use! To be honest, because I wanted results, I loved the hardest ones. Chief and Em introduced me to exercises I'd never done on my own, and it's amazing how much this affected my overall fitness and core strength.

Which exercise did you dread the most?

I still dread treadmill intervals. The incline is cranked and when you are hurting you can't slow it down, like you can on a bike or cross trainer. I must say, though, I think this is what got rid of that last layer of chub for me.

Did you discover any new favourite foods?

Lots of healthy options like konjac rice. Also bread from the Protein Bread Co. really helped with the carb cravings.

How did you stay motivated on hard days?

I made it a part of my job. As far as time goes, you really do have to make a commitment. Chief and Em said we had to strive for 5 sessions a week. I made a decision to MAKE it happen. Sometimes that meant working out at 11pm, or in a hotel gym if I was away. But I shocked myself by exercising 7 times a week.

What is your top tip for someone just starting?

Dive in. If you go hard straight away and REALLY stick to a strict diet, you will see results quickly, which will inspire you to keep going. You'll shock yourself and be so proud. It gets easier. If you go half-arsed, the results take longer to kick in and you'll probably give up. If chubby, time-poor me can do it, you can too!

TRANSFORMATION STORIES
JULES'S STORY

Name: Jules Sebastian

Age: 38

Occupation: Presenter, Stylist & Wellness Ambassador

When did you complete the 8WTW program? Mid 2017

What motivated you to undertake this program?

I'd kind of given up on my health and fitness. I made every excuse under the sun (two kids, too busy, no time) not to exercise and as a result, my body was really soft. I wasn't paying attention to what I was eating because I was of the mindset that I couldn't do anything about it. I didn't feel good about myself, I was conscious that I had a few extra kg's, my clothes were really tight and I had a constant headache and a negative attitude. When my husband came home and told me he'd met with some trainers and that we were starting to train tomorrow, I had a choice: either refuse, or take control of my situation and commit myself to trying. I did the latter and haven't looked back!

What goals did you set for yourself?

I didn't know what to expect. My goals were very basic – it was just to give it a go to see if I could do it. I was so unsure of what I was capable of!

Did you meet those goals?

I exceeded far above anything I thought possible! I'm floored by the results. My body literally transformed.

Which aspect of the program did you find the most challenging?

The diet! I went into autopilot on the exercise front: I'd get up, put on gym clothes, drop the kids at school and head to the gym. But the food took up all my brain space. I had to grocery shop differently and make healthier choices for every snack and meal.

Which week was the hardest for you? Why?

Week 2. My muscles were on fire and I was finding it hard to walk and get dressed! I had sugar withdrawals and huge headaches. I truly wanted to give up – all the trying seemed for nothing. But by Week 3, I was stronger physically, so I wasn't as sore. I'd also kicked my sugar addiction, and was suddenly experiencing the healthy high I'd heard about.

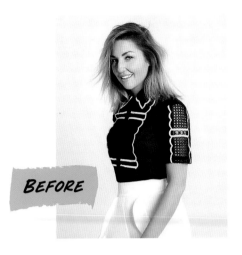

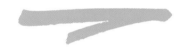
BEFORE

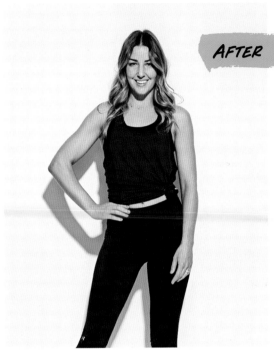
AFTER

EM AND CHIEF ARE LEGENDS. I NOW KNOW EXACTLY WHAT TO DO IN THE GYM AND IN THE GROCERY STORE.

Favourite exercise from the workouts?

Favourite?! Definitely no favourites, but I didn't mind the resistance work we did. Chief had me doing biceps and shoulders with the barbells. My weights went up weekly and I felt really strong by the end of the 8 weeks. My arms were ripped too!

Which exercise did you dread the most?

By far the ropes. It's the cardio/resistance combo that makes you so tired. Em was relentless and by the last set I was always yelling at her! It gave great all-over results though, so I'm glad I persevered.

Did you discover any new favourite foods?

So many. I discovered a love for vegies of all types. When you take out all the artificial stuff from your diet and get down to natural options, you can taste all sorts of good things in each bite. I thought I'd miss bad food much more than I actually do. Turns out I'm also one of those people who really love kale!

How did you stay motivated on hard days?

It was really motivating to have Guy alongside me working towards a healthy life. On the days it was hard, I had to remember what I was doing it for: feeling amazing, looking better and having endless energy. I felt so proud of myself for sticking to it and not giving up. That in itself encouraged me to keep going.

What is your top tip for someone just starting?

Do it! Prioritise your health. We have one body, and one life to live. I'm just like any other busy, working parent. It's not easy for any of us to fit everything into a day. When I say this changed my life, it's not an overstatement. Since making my health a priority, I worry less, my anxiety has dropped, I'm more focused at work and happier to be with my kids at home. I also seem to fit more into a day (which I can't believe). My overall attitude is positive. If that's not enough reason to start, I don't know what is!

THE
LIST //

THE KETO
KICKSTART

When you begin the 8WTW program and eat only the foods on The List, you will have removed practically all of the sugar from your everyday diet. Hopefully, you will experience ketosis, which means your body has switched to burning fat as its main fuel source. The idea isn't to stay in ketosis – most people might only be at that point for a few days or a week at most. It's what we call a 'keto kickstart' to carb-conscious living – the 8WTW transformation.

We will then spend the next 8 weeks building up to a plate full of the nutrients that you need as a properly functioning human being. You absolutely cannot be on a restricted 'diet' for your entire life. Not only is it miserable, it isn't healthy. Following the 8WTW program for 8 weeks is the best way to get your body back to understanding food as fuel, and giving it the best and healthiest fuel that you can. If you do this properly, you can have the foods you miss once the 8 weeks are done. By then, you will have learned

to enjoy healthier foods and smaller portions – you'll understand that moderation is key to everything.

The aim of your daily food intake is to spread it out so that you eat every 2–3 hours at the very least. We want to keep your metabolism at its peak. If you haven't treated your body well and are used to eating only once or twice a day, you need to speed up your metabolism by eating regularly and often.

On the first 2–3 days of the 8WTW program, you may feel some side effects, such as light-headedness, slight headaches or weakness. However, about 70% of people don't experience any of these symptoms – they are the people who already have a relatively clean way of eating. Those who drink a lot of coffee, eat a lot of processed foods or high sugar foods (including dried fruits, sports drinks, fizzy drinks and sugar in general) are going to really feel the change. But don't give up! Push through and maybe have

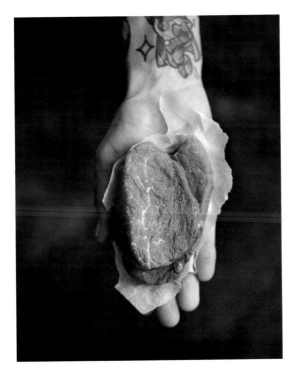

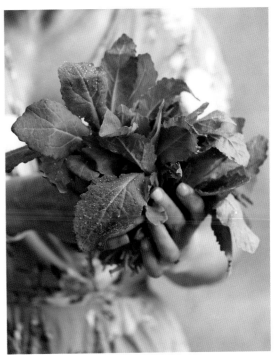

a Berocca or vitamin B supplement and go a little easier in your training, but don't give up. This phase needs to occur in order for you to move through to the next phase and kickstart your body into burning fat.

You are only human and you are going to want to eat and drink things that aren't on this plan. But stick with it – you will feel amazing once you get the hang of making healthier choices. If you can go a week without chocolate, you will change everything!

And remember, ladies: you don't need as much food as a man. One of the biggest mistakes a woman can make is to eat the same portion size as the man in her life. Male or female, your protein and carbohydrate portions should be the size of your palm.

YOU ARE ONLY HUMAN AND YOU ARE GOING TO WANT TO EAT AND DRINK THINGS THAT AREN'T ON THIS PLAN. BUT STICK WITH IT – YOU WILL FEEL AMAZING ONCE YOU GET THE HANG OF MAKING HEALTHIER CHOICES.

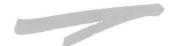

WATER

Water is one of the most important aspects of the program, because it flushes out toxins and will make you feel better when you hit an energy slump.

Drinking enough water can be a hard habit to follow, especially when you grow tired of running to the bathroom every half an hour. But don't let this habit fall by the wayside. You need to drink a minimum of 2 litres (70 fl oz/8 cups) of water a day for your body to function properly (more when you're working out), so this is not negotiable.

If you fall off the track with your water intake, you need to get back onto this pronto – tell yourself that of all the changes you're making, this is the most important.

Water makes up close to 70% of your body, and even more of your organs. The liver alone is 85% water. What does your liver do? It breaks down toxins and removes them, but it simply can't do that without water. Your liver breaks down all the fatty acids in your food and transports them to your bloodstream to be metabolised. When you cut back on water or replace it with alternatives, your poor old kidneys (whose job is also to remove toxins and waste) don't work properly. And then, because your kidneys are not doing their job, your liver picks up the slack and it can't do its job of metabolising fat. So everything slows down, which is the opposite of what you want to be happening, especially while on the 8WTW program. That's why water consumption is so important, not to mention the fact that 2 litres of water a day can take years off your face and body. A properly hydrated human looks about a hundred times healthier than one who is thirsty or living on drinks that are diuretics (i.e. caffeinated and sugary drinks). Convinced yet?

ALCOHOL

Let's talk about alcohol. While some people can easily turn that switch off and not even think about drinking for the entire 8 weeks, others find it much harder. Alcohol might be your little vice, or a social crutch that makes you feel more relaxed and easy-going around colleagues and friends. Perhaps you drink when entertaining clients or guests, or alcohol is just something you've become used to having every evening. Whatever your reasons, we want you to understand why you'll get better results from the 8WTW program without alcohol. (If you aren't a drinker, you won't need to think about this at all. Too easy!)

There's a simple reason why you need to avoid all alcohol while you're on the program: alcohol will SABOTAGE your best efforts on this training program. Once you get through the 8 weeks, it's an entirely different story – your body and mind will be transformed by then, so if you want to, you can reintroduce alcohol into your diet. The odd drink isn't the end of the world. But before that can happen, we need to reboot your metabolism and set up your new physique. Life is for living, but there's no sense in going overboard in any one area. Dial everything back to moderation – that includes alcohol.

Once it enters your body, alcohol breaks down very differently to food and other drinks. When you drink alcohol, your body reacts to it as a toxin so it's quickly diffused through your stomach lining and into your bloodstream, where it travels to your liver and brain. Now, here's the important part: if there's alcohol in your system, your liver will attend to it first, and give it priority over anything else. This means that the rest of your body can't concentrate on properly breaking down the ordinary stuff like carbs, fats and proteins. This in turn makes the body store these nutrients as body fat – usually on the parts of your body where you least want it.

Some of our 8WTW followers have asked why they get tipsy or drunk so much faster when they're being healthy, and even more so if they have an empty stomach. This is because the more alcohol you push into your liver (which can be processed from the glass in a matter of minutes), the harder it has to work. Since your liver can only cope with little bits at a time, it pushes the rest away and it floats around your body (in your blood and in your brain), making you feel drunk.

Another important thing to note is that there is no nutritional value in alcohol (no, it doesn't count as fruit!). Alcoholic drinks are nothing but empty calories, and if you are working so hard at sticking

to The List and getting your training in 6 days a week, why set yourself back by downing hundreds of empty calories in one drink?

Personally, I think the reason that drinking is so damaging when you're working towards a goal is that it affects the part of your brain that makes logical decisions. It turns your goals into tomorrow's problem. When this happens, that late-night trip to KFC or a Chinese take-away is much more likely.

We aren't saying you can't enjoy the odd glass of wine or beer once you've completed your 8 weeks. It all comes back to that key word: moderation. And appreciating that the drink in your hand is not the last drink you'll ever have.

MORE ON THE NEXT PAGE »

THE LIST *AT A GLANCE*

To make life easy for you, we've pulled together this overview so you can remind yourself quickly of the foods you're able to eat over the next 8 weeks. We go into more detail about The List in the individual weeks, but these are the pages you can come back to whenever you're standing in the kitchen, or sitting in a restaurant wondering, 'What can I eat?' It's a good idea to snap a photo of these pages so you always have it handy when you're out and about, or make a few photocopies to stick up in your kitchen or office – wherever you need to see it.

COMPULSORY GREENS

 150 g (5½ oz) every day

200 g (7 oz) every day

+ Baby English spinach
+ Celery (unlimited)
+ Cucumber (unlimited)
+ Lettuce (all types)
+ Watercress

VEGETABLES

 150 g (5½ oz) every day

200 g (7 oz) every day

+ Asparagus
+ Avocado (only ¼ per day)
+ Bean sprouts
+ Bok choy (pak choy)
+ Capsicum (pepper)
+ Chinese cabbage (wong bok)
+ Eggplant (aubergine)
+ English spinach (fresh or frozen)
+ Fennel

+ Mushrooms
+ Okra
+ Onion
+ Radish
+ Spring onion (scallion)
+ Tomato (no more than ½ medium tomato or 6 cherry tomatoes per day)
+ Zucchini (courgette)

IN WEEK 3, INCREASE THE DAILY SERVING SIZE (SEE PAGE 94) AND START TO ADD IN

+ Broccoli
+ Brussels sprouts
+ Cabbage
+ Carrot
+ Cauliflower
+ Leek
+ Pumpkin (winter squash)
+ Runner beans
+ Squash
+ String beans

IN WEEK 7 START TO ADD IN

+ Sweet potato (as an alternative to one portion of grains)

MEATS AND SEAFOOD

A serve is a palm-sized portion of protein per meal. You can have 3 serves per day.

+ Beef: lean cuts, veal or minced* (ground)
+ Chicken: lean meat or minced* (ground) only – no skin, no wings, no stuffing, not fried, no sauce (Nando's or Oporto chicken with no sauce is fine).
+ Fish: fresh, frozen or tinned (if tinned, in springwater or brine only)
+ Kangaroo and kangaroo sausages
+ Lamb: very lean cuts
+ Pork: very lean cuts, including low-fat ham, trimmed bacon and shoulder bacon
+ Seafood: any fresh, frozen or tinned (in springwater or brine only), including shellfish and crustaceans
+ Smoked salmon
+ Turkey: lean meat or minced* (ground) only – no skin or wings

*Minced (ground) meats must be under 8% fat.

DAIRY AND EGGS

+ Cheeses: only fat-free or very low-fat cheese products (no more than 30 g/1 oz per day)
+ Egg whites (unlimited)
+ Egg yolks (no more than 2 per day)
+ Milk: skim or fat-free/non-fat (up to 300 ml/10½ fl oz per day)
+ Non-dairy milks: unsweetened low-fat or skim soy milk or unsweetened almond milk (up to 300 ml/10½ fl oz per day)
+ Sour cream: only fat-free or very low fat (no more than 30 g/1 oz per day)
+ Yoghurt: 1 serve per day of low-fat, low-carb, low-sugar plain or vanilla yoghurt (under 6 g sugar per serve)

GET EXCITED ABOUT THESE FOODS. THEY HAVE THE POWER TO CHANGE YOUR LIFE.

STRICTLY OFF LIMITS!

Getting your head around what is OFF the list is just as important as knowing what's on it. Alcohol (in any form) is a no-go, as are these things: butter, margarine, fried foods and 'treat foods' like ice cream, frozen yoghurt, pies, pastries, cakes – you get the idea. Junk foods (there are way too many to list here) like biscuits, chips, dips, chocolate and the like are also firmly off-limits, as are any oils not specified on this list (this includes extra virgin oil in salad dressings and other cooking oils).

BREADS, NOODLES AND GRAINS

You can have 1 serve per day

+ 2 slices of Protein bread from The Protein Bread Co. (theproteinbreadco.com.au)
+ 1 pizza base from The Protein Bread Co. (go easy on the cheese)
+ Konjac, shirataki or Slendier noodles (found in the health food aisle of the supermarket and Asian grocery stores)
+ Konjac rice

ON WEEKENDS STARTING IN WEEK 4, ADD

1 portion of grains (or corn) from the list below on whichever day you aren't eating fruit.

 ½ cup cooked grains or corn

 ⅔ cup cooked grains or corn (1 cup if you are over 183 cm/6 ft tall)

+ Brown rice
+ Buckwheat
+ Couscous (any kind)
+ Gluten-free pasta
+ Lentils
+ Oats
+ Quinoa
+ Wild rice
+ Corn (fresh)

IN WEEK 7 YOU CAN START ADDING

1 portion of grains 3 times a week (with a day in between)

FRUIT

ON THE WEEKEND OF WEEK 4, ADD FRUIT

Choose one day (the day that is going to be grain free) and have 1 serve of fruit that day.

+ Apples (1 medium)
+ Apricots (2 small)
+ Bananas (1 medium)
+ Blackberries (½ cup)
+ Blueberries (½ cup)
+ Cherries (1 cup)
+ Cranberries (½ cup)
+ Grapes (1 cup)
+ Honeydew melon (1 slice)
+ Mandarins (1 small)
+ Mango (1 cup)
+ Nectarines (1 small)
+ Peaches (1 small)
+ Raspberries (½ cup)
+ Strawberries (½ cup)
+ Watermelon (1 slice)

THEN, STARTING IN WEEK 5 YOU CAN HAVE 1 SERVE OF FRUIT EVERY OTHER DAY.

HERBS, SPICES AND OTHER KEY INGREDIENTS

+ Black pepper (freshly ground)
+ Canola oil spray (use sparingly, and not in all recipes)
+ Chia seeds
+ Chilli: fresh red/green chilli, chilli flakes, ancho chilli, smoked chipotle chilli
+ Chlorophyll (best in liquid form and very important for a healthy gut)
+ Curry paste and powder
+ Dried spices (essentials are paprika, roast vegetable seasoning and Asian spice blends)
+ French shallots
+ Garlic
+ Ginger
+ Herbs: as many as you like, fresh or dried
+ Lemon
+ Lemongrass
+ Lime
+ Linseed (flaxseed) oil
+ Mustard
+ Nori sheets
+ Protein powder
+ Salt-reduced soy sauce
+ Sea salt
+ Stock: low-sodium liquid stock and stock (bouillon) cubes
+ Sugar-free chewing gum
+ Sugar-free non-fat cocoa powder
+ Sugar-free sweeteners: e.g. stevia, Splenda, Equal (use as little as possible)
+ Tabasco sauce
+ Vanilla extract
+ Vinegar: apple cider, balsamic, white
+ Vitamin B supplement or Berocca

IN WEEK 3, START ADDING IN
+ Coconut oil (1 teaspoon per day)
+ Natural almonds every second day (15 for women and 20 for men)

DRINKS

+ Water (up to 3 litres/105 fl oz/12 cups per day)
+ Coffee (up to 3 per day if made with water, only 1 per day if made with milk)
+ Tea and herbal tea (up to 3 per day)
+ Fresh ginger tea
+ Sugar-free hot chocolate (only 1 per day)

RECIPES AND THE LIST

Very occasionally, a recipe in this book might include an ingredient that isn't on The List (like the tomato paste used in the Eggplant Lasagne on page 162). This doesn't mean it's OK for you to start cooking with tomato paste again, it just means that – for that one recipe – you get a pass.

THE
DARC
WORKOU

TS//

WANT IT?
EARN IT!

The first fallacy I want to dismiss is the commonly held belief that achieving your health and fitness goals is '80% nutrition and 20% training'. This misconception is one of the biggest things holding you back. No matter how well you eat, unless you focus on the quality and consistency of your training, you will never get stronger, fitter, faster or more toned. As you will quickly learn, the 8WTW program is based on the principle that results come from a 50/50 balance of the two.

Over the past 25 plus years I've had the opportunity to learn from some of the greatest minds in exercise science, athletic performance, and strength and conditioning from right around the world. I have taken this wealth of knowledge and interpreted it in order to create a highly effective, time-efficient training regime that achieves dramatic results in just 8 weeks. Even more important, when combined with Emilie's carb-conscious eating program, these results can be maintained long term without letting calorie-counting rule your life.

The second thing I want you to understand is that results come from hard work. There are no shortcuts or cheats. Put simply, the more you put into your

training, the more you'll get out of it. Don't let that thought dissuade you from committing to this program, though. Nothing about the training we are going to take you through is beyond you. You just need to put in your own best effort every time you train.

WELCOME TO THE DARCSIDE

At the heart of the 8WTW training philosophy is what's known as the DARC Protocol. DARC stands for Dynamic, Aerobic, Resisted Conditioning. All you really need to know is that DARC has been designed to shred fat, increase athleticism and improve muscle tone all at the same time.

Part of the reason that DARC training is so effective is due to the fact it is a hybrid of a number of proven training techniques, arranged in a manner that makes every second, and every rep, of your workout count towards your overall goal.

Let me break it down for you. Every session you do throughout this program will combine resistance training with high intensity interval training (HIIT). Most people looking to achieve fat loss have heard about HIIT over the past couple of years but, unfortunately, the majority are doing it wrong.

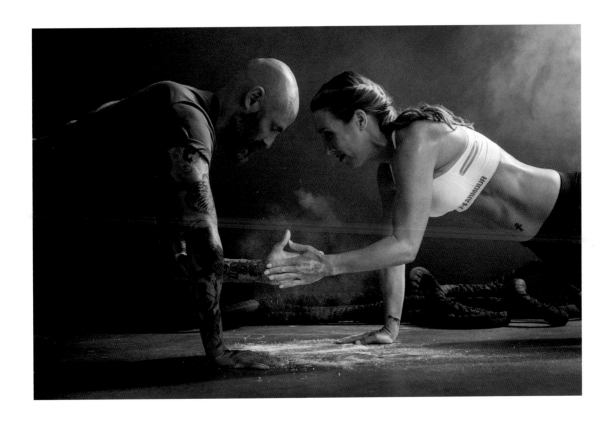

When it comes to HIIT, the single most important element is intensity.

Most individuals who come to train with Em, myself or our team are already training, whether it be on their own, with another trainer or in a group. The fact that they have taken the initiative to contact us usually means that what they are currently doing just isn't working.

Traditionally, programs would prescribe separate cardio sessions (possibly HIIT) and strength sessions. However, from a fat-burning perspective, if a whole 45-minute session is based purely on cardio, by the end of the workout the level of intensity is far lower than we would hope for.

On the other hand, when most people are doing strength-based workouts, they tend to spend the majority of their time resting between sets. To give you some insight, most professionally designed weight training programs only see you lifting less than 17% of the time. The rest of the workout is spent resting in preparation for the next set.

The theory behind DARC training is surprisingly simple. Use the time spent doing strength work to recover from your bouts of HIIT in order to be able to maintain the intensity all the way through to the end of the workout. And use the time doing those bouts of HIIT to fill the periods of recovery between strength sets, which most people spend looking at their mobile phones, watching TV or socialising.

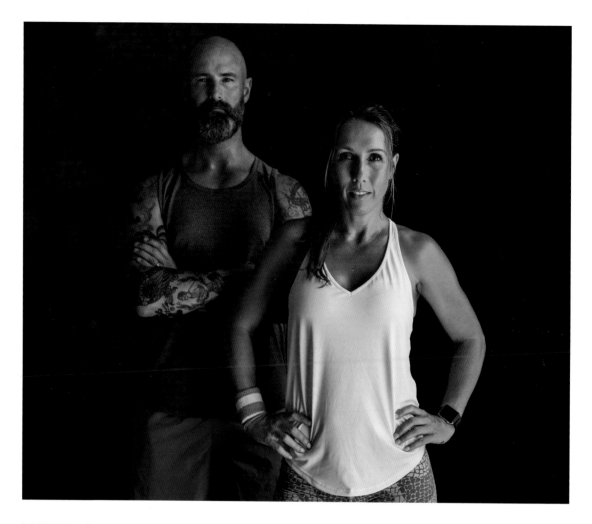

Let's get started

As you read through this section, you will notice that I've broken each week down into four separate workouts, each focusing on two to three different muscle groups. Each workout consists of three parts or mini-circuits. Each circuit is made up of two strength exercises and one conditioning (or cardio) exercise. The key to getting the best results from each DARC workout is to CHALLENGE yourself on each and every set. On the strength exercises, don't rest for too long at the top or bottom of the movement. Try to maintain a consistent cadence. When it comes to the conditioning exercises, be sure to keep up the pace, and to push as hard as you can (without losing form) for the last 10 seconds of every set. Get it done!

DAY 1:
DAYS TO WOW: *56*

WORKING ON:
LEGS, GLUTES, ABS

→ DAY ONE: PART ONE →

Goblet squats
40sec ON / 20sec REST

[1] Stand with your feet hip-width apart. Lace your fingers together at chin height with your elbows pointing straight down. [2] Keeping your weight on your heels, sit down as deep as possible, until your elbows are between your knees. [3] Drive down hard through your heels and stand back up straight.

Jackknives
40sec ON / 20sec REST

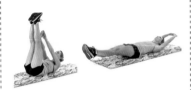

[1] Lie on your back, bend your knees and bring your legs up as straight as possible, then reach up for your ankles. [2] From here, slowly lower your hands and feet towards the ground, stopping just before you touch (this should take 4sec). [3] Slowly squeeze back to the top, focusing on pulling up through your toes (again this should take 4sec).

Upper-body jumping jacks
20sec ON / 10sec REST

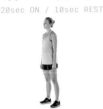 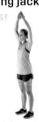

[1] Stand with your feet slightly apart, your knees unlocked and your arms by your sides. [2] Keeping your arms straight, swing them out to the sides and straight up above your head until your hands touch. [3] Swing your arms back down until your palms slap the outside of your thighs.

> **Repeat this exercise but for 20sec on and 60sec rest.**

→ DAY ONE: PART TWO →

Bulgarian split squat
20sec ON / 10sec REST

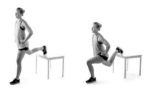

[1] Stand one stride in front of a chair or low table, then lift up your right foot, reach back and put your toes on the chair. [2] With your hands resting on your hips, bend your left knee and lower yourself down, pushing your right knee back towards the chair. [3] Now press down through your left heel and drive up until your left knee is straight.

> **Repeat this exercise with the right leg.**

Supine window washers
40sec ON / 20sec REST

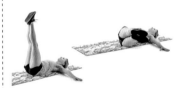

[1] Lie on your back with your arms stretched out to the sides, palms down. [2] Bend your knees and bring your legs up as straight as possible. [3] Slowly lower your legs down to the left, stopping just short of the floor, then slowly bring your legs back up until they are directly over your hips. [4] Repeat, lowering your legs down to the right.

Upper-body cross countries
20sec ON / 10sec REST

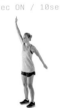 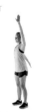

[1] Stand with your feet slightly apart and your knees unlocked. [2] Swing your right arm forward as high as possible as you swing your left arm back as far as possible. [3] Now swing your arms through as fast as possible until your left arm is above your head to the front, and your right arm is stretched back behind you.

> **Repeat this exercise but for 20sec on and 60sec rest.**

Supine hamstring curl
20sec ON / 10sec REST

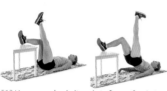

[1] Lie on your back directly in front of a chair or low table with your right knee bent and your right heel on the chair. Straighten your left leg. [2] Push down as hard as you can through your right heel, squeezing your glutes. Your hips will start to rise up off the floor. [3] Hold at the top of the movement for a two-count, then slowly lower your hips back down.

Repeat this exercise with the left leg.

Low-profile sit-ups
40sec ON / 20sec REST

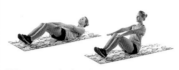

[1] Lie on your back with your knees bent at 90 degrees and your hands beside your thighs. [2] Squeeze your rib cage towards your pelvis and reach forward until your thumbs are alongside your kneecaps. [3] Slowly lower your shoulders back down towards the floor.

Upper-body SEAL jacks
20sec ON / 10sec REST

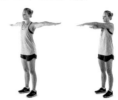

[1] Stand with your feet hip-width apart and your arms stretched straight out to the sides, palms down, at shoulder level. [2] Keeping your arms at shoulder level, swing them forward until your elbows cross in front of you. [3] Next, again keeping your arms up at shoulder level, swing them back as far as possible.

Repeat this exercise but for 20sec on and 60sec rest.

DAY 2:
DAYS TO WOW: 55

WORKING ON:
CHEST, BACK

Repeat 3 Rounds

Deep push-ups
20sec ON / 10sec REST

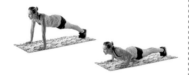

[1] Take up the military push-up position with your hands shoulder-width apart and your feet together. [2] Keeping your body locked tight, slowly lower your chest towards the floor. [3] Once your chest touches the floor, push down hard through the heels of your palms, driving back up until your elbows are straight.

Supine elbow push-ups
20sec ON / 10sec REST

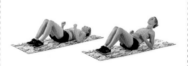

[1] Lie on your back with your knees and elbows bent at 90 degrees and your arms at a 45-degree angle from your body. [2] Press down through your elbows as hard as you can, lifting your shoulder blades up off the ground. [3] Slowly lower yourself back down to the floor.

Squat jumps
20sec ON / 10sec REST

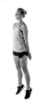

[1] Stand with your feet hip-width apart. [2] Sit down into a deep squat with your weight on your heels and your arms stretched out in front of you. [3] Drive down through your heels and leap up tall. [4] Land with bent knees and drop straight down into the next squat.

Repeat this exercise but for 20sec on and 60sec rest.

Decline push-ups

20sec ON / 10sec REST

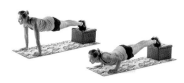

[1] Take up the standard push-up position, with your toes up on a low stool or similar. [2] Keeping your body locked, lower your chest towards the ground. [3] Push down hard through the heels of your palms and drive back up until your elbows are straight.

NOTE: To reduce the intensity, rest your knees on the stool instead of your toes.

Downward dog to cobra

20sec ON / 10sec REST

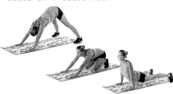

[1] Take up the standard push-up position. Move your feet shoulder-width apart, push your hips up high and walk your hands back towards your feet until you're looking straight back through your knees. [2] Now, bend your knees, lowering them until they are about 2.5 cm (1 inch) from the floor. [3] Push your hips forward and down until they are 2.5 cm (1 inch) from the floor. Your elbows should be straight, and your chest up tall. [4] Reverse the movement until you are back in the original downward dog position.

Switch lunges

20sec ON / 10sec REST

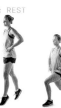

[1] Stand with your feet hip-width apart and your hands on your hips. Take a big step forward with your right foot. You should now be up on your back toes. [2] Lower your back knee down towards the ground, then drive up and switch your legs so that your left leg is now in front. [3] Lower your back knee down towards the ground, then drive up and switch your legs again.

Repeat this exercise but for 20sec on and 60sec rest.

Close-grip push-ups

20sec ON / 10sec REST

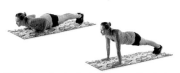

[1] Take up the standard push-up position, but place your hands down a little closer to your hips than usual. [2] As you lower yourself down towards the ground, leading with your chest, your elbows should slide tightly past your rib cage. [3] Once your chest touches the ground, push down hard through the heels of your palms and drive back up until your elbows are straight.

Doorframe rows

20sec ON / 10sec REST

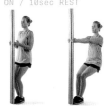

[1] Stand in a doorway with your toes touching the doorframe and your knees slightly bent, gripping the doorframe with both hands. [2] Keeping your heels on the ground, lock your body, extend your arms and lean back. [3] Now, keeping your body locked straight, drag your elbows back past your ribs, pulling yourself towards the doorframe. [4] When your knees are almost touching the doorframe, pause for a second before extending your arms and slowly lowering yourself backwards again.

Switch squats

20sec ON / 10sec REST

[1] Stand with your feet 5 cm (2 inches) apart, toes straight ahead. [2] Sit into a deep squat with your weight on your heels and your arms out in front. [3] Drive down through your heels and leap up tall, landing with your heels wide and your toes at 45 degrees. [4] Sit into a sumo squat, keeping your knees in line with your toes, then leap up and land in the original position.

Repeat this exercise but for 20sec on and 60sec rest.

NOTE: WHEN DOING PUSH-UPS, IF YOU'RE UNABLE TO COME BACK UP ON YOUR TOES, PUT YOUR KNEES ON THE GROUND AS YOU PUSH UP, THEN RETURN TO YOUR TOES BEFORE YOU LOWER AGAIN.

DAY 3:
DAYS TO WOW: *54*

WORKING ON:
BICEPS, TRICEPS

→ DAY THREE: PART ONE →

Doorframe bicep curls
20sec ON / 10sec REST

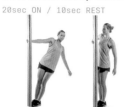

[1] Stand in a doorway, facing the doorframe. Lift your right arm up to shoulder level and clasp the edge of the doorframe with your fingertips. [2] Keeping your elbow at shoulder level, lock your body and bend your elbow, pulling your right shoulder towards the doorframe. [3] Slowly straighten your arm and push yourself back to the start position.

Repeat this exercise on the left side.

Tricep dips
20sec ON / 10sec REST

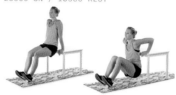

[1] Push a chair or low table up against something to stop it from moving. Sit on the edge of the chair with your palms flat and your thumbs under the edge of your butt. [2] Take your weight onto your hands, sliding your hips forward off the edge of the chair. [3] Bend your elbows and lower your butt towards the floor, keeping your back as close to the chair as possible. [4] When you can't get any lower, push down hard through your hands and drive back up until your elbows are straight.

Mountain climbers
20sec ON / 10sec REST

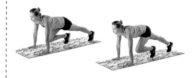

[1] Take up the standard push-up position. Keeping your body locked, bring your right knee up towards your chest and rest your toe on the floor. [2] Keeping tight through your mid-section, push off your right foot and switch legs so that your left knee is pulled up towards your chest. [3] Push off your left foot and switch legs again.

Repeat this exercise but for 20sec on and 60sec rest.

→ DAY THREE: PART TWO →

Seated towel curls
20sec ON / 10sec REST

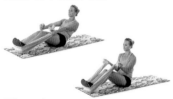

[1] Sit on the ground with your knees bent at 90 degrees. [2] Hook a bath towel over your feet and grip both ends of the towel. [3] With your palms facing up, slowly straighten your arms, lowering your shoulders towards the floor. [4] Now, bend your elbows as if you are trying to touch your knuckles to your collarbone. Try to push your weight back through your shoulders in order to create as much resistance as possible.

Badger push-ups
20sec ON / 10sec REST

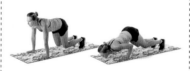

[1] Take up the table-top position, with your hands directly under your shoulders and knees directly under your hips. Push down into the floor with your toes so that your knees are 2.5 cm (1 inch) off the ground. [2] Sit back on your haunches, with your butt resting on your calves. [3] Bend your elbows and aim to touch your chin on the ground between your fingertips. [4] Leading with your hips, push down hard through your palms and drive back until your butt is resting on your calves again.

Frogs
20sec ON / 10sec REST

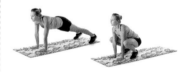

[1] Take up the standard push-up position. Drive down hard through your toes and pull your knees up either side of your elbows until you are in the frog position. [2] Shift your weight back over your hands and kick back out into the push-up position again.

Repeat this exercise but for 20sec on and 60sec rest.

Leg-resisted hammer curl
20sec ON / 10sec REST

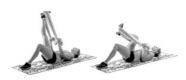

[1] Lie on your back, hook a bath towel over your right foot and grip both ends of the towel. [2] Push your foot up while resisting with your arms. [3] Once your arms are straight, bend your elbows and fold your arms as if you are trying to touch your thumbs to your shoulders. At the same time, keep tension on the towel with your foot and don't let your arms fold.

Repeat this exercise on the left side.

Diamond push-ups
20sec ON / 10sec REST

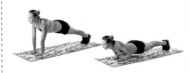

[1] Take up the standard push-up position, but bring your hands together under your chest, creating a diamond shape with your index fingers and thumbs. Your hands need to be a little lower than the standard push-up position. [2] Bend your elbows and lower yourself down until your chest touches the back of your hands. [3] Now, keeping your body locked, push down hard through your palms and drive back up until your elbows are straight.

Squat thrust
20sec ON / 10sec REST

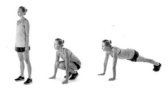

[1] Stand up straight with your feet hip-width apart. [2] Drop down until your butt is resting on the back of your calves, with your hands on the floor. [3] Shift your weight over your hands and kick out into a push-up position. [4] Jump back into the crouch position, with your knees between your elbows. [5] Drive down through your heels and stand up tall.

Repeat this exercise but for 20sec on and 60sec rest.

DAY 4:
DAYS TO WOW: 53

WORKING ON:
SHOULDERS, ABS

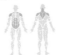

Repeat
3
Rounds

Shoulder push-ups
20sec ON / 10sec REST

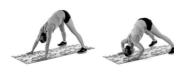

[1] Take up the standard push-up position. Move your feet out to shoulder width, push your hips up high and walk your hands back towards your feet until you're looking straight back through your knees. Turn your fingers in slightly. [2] Slowly bend your elbows and lower yourself down, aiming to touch the top of your head gently on the ground between your hands. [3] Push down hard through your palms and drive back up until your elbows are straight.

Stutter sit-ups
40sec ON / 20sec REST

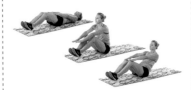

[1] Start in the standard military sit-up position, with your knees bent at 90 degrees and your hands resting on your thighs. [2] Squeeze your rib cage towards your pelvis, sliding your hands along your thighs until your elbows are resting on your knees. [3] Slowly lower yourself back until your palms are resting on your knees, but your back is still off the ground. [4] Squeeze back up until your elbows are back on your knees. [5] Lower back down to the start position.

Speed skaters
20sec ON / 10sec REST

[1] Stand with your feet hip-width apart. [2] Leap as wide to the left as possible, landing on your left foot and swinging your right leg behind your left. [3] Swing your right leg back out to the right, leaping as wide as possible and landing on your right foot, swinging your left leg behind your right leg.

Repeat this exercise but for 20sec on and 60sec rest.

Hindu push-ups

20sec ON / 10sec REST

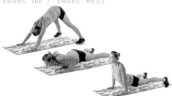

[1] Take up the standard push-up position, but have your feet shoulder-width apart and your hips as high in the air as possible. [2] Bend your elbows and lower yourself as if you are going to touch your forehead to the ground between your hands. Before it touches, slide your body forward as if you are going to touch your nose, then chin, chest and hips in the same spot. [3] Once your hips are in line with your hands, arch your back and straighten your elbows. [4] Lift your hips as high as possible and push into the start position.

Push-up position hold

40sec ON / 20sec REST

[1] Take up the standard military push-up position. [2] Hold this position for the prescribed time, ensuring you keep a straight line between your shoulders, hips and ankles.

> NOTE: Be careful not to drop or lift your hips.

High jumps

20sec ON / 10sec REST

[1] Stand with your feet hip-width apart. [2] Sit into a half-squat with your arms in front of you. [3] Swing your arms back past your hips, leaping up as high as possible. At the same time, draw your knees up towards your chest until you are in a tuck position in midair. [4] Land with bent knees and drop straight down into the next half-squat.

> Repeat this exercise but for 20sec on and 60sec rest.

Cross-body ankle taps

20sec ON / 10sec REST

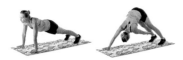

[1] Take up the standard push-up position, with your feet shoulder-width apart. [2] Drive your hips upwards, then pick up your left hand and reach through to tap your right ankle. [3] Lower yourself back down to a dead-straight push-up position. [4] Drive your hips back up, then pick up your right hand and reach through to tap your left ankle. [5] Return to a dead-straight push-up position.

Overhead sit-ups

40sec ON / 20sec REST

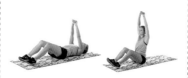

[1] Start in the standard military sit-up position, with your knees bent at 90 degrees and your arms straight up as if you are reaching for the ceiling. [2] Squeeze your rib cage towards your hips and drive up into a seated position. Your arms should still be stretched up towards the sky. [3] Slowly lower yourself back down to the start position.

Toe taps

20sec ON / 10sec REST

[1] Stand in front of a step or something similar that is about 20 cm (8 inches) high. [2] Rest the bottom of your right toes on the edge of the step, with your weight on your left leg. [3] Jump up and switch legs so that you are standing on your right leg, with your left toes resting on the step.

> Repeat this exercise but for 20sec on and 60sec rest.

GREAT WORK! THE FIRST STEPS ARE ALWAYS THE HARDEST. KEEP GOING.

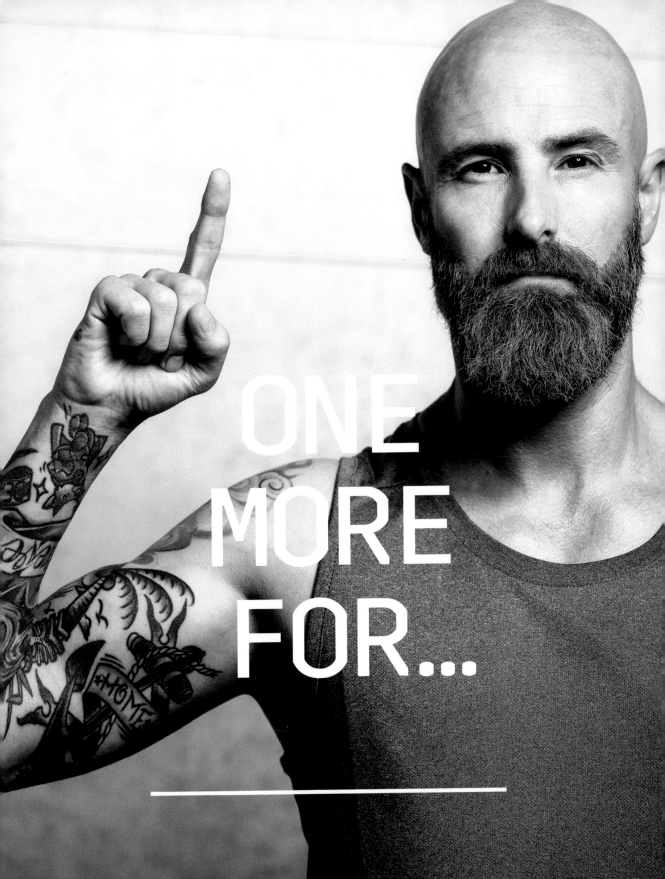

ONE
MORE
FOR...

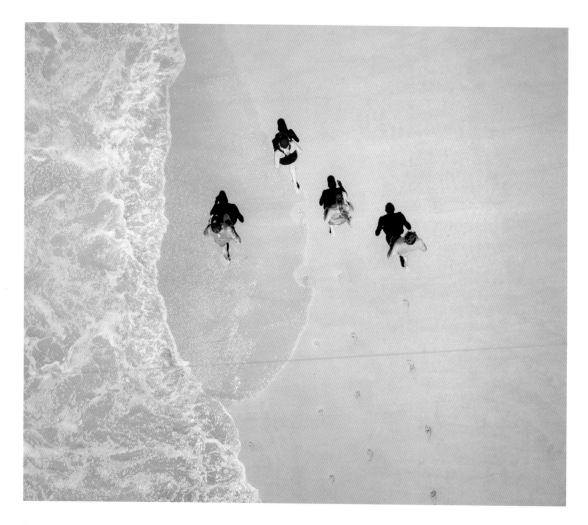

WEEKS 3–4
Time to take it up a gear

Over the last 2 weeks, we have built a strong base, and you will undoubtedly have already seen and felt some serious improvements. Now is the time to make the most of that momentum, so we are going to add a few more challenging exercises to your repertoire. As always, you should focus on form over speed. This will not only help you avoid injury, but will also ensure that you get the most out of every workout. Just remember, the better your form, the better the results. By now you should be quite adept at pushing as hard as possible during those final 10 seconds of each set on the conditioning exercises. Keep up that intensity, and try to challenge yourself to get more reps done each time.

DAY 1:
DAYS TO WOW: *42*

WORKING ON:
LEGS, GLUTES, ABS

Repeat
3
Rounds

→ DAY ONE: **PART ONE** →

Stutter squats
40sec ON / 20sec REST

[1] Stand with your feet hip-width apart, hands by your sides. [2] Leading with your glutes, sit into a deep squat, reaching forward with your arms in order to stay balanced. Your goal is to get your butt to the back of your calves (or as close as possible). [3] Come halfway up, until your thighs are parallel to the ground. [4] Lower back down again, then drive all the way back up to a standing position.

Pocket knives
40sec ON / 20sec REST

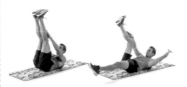

[1] Lie on your back, bend your knees and bring your legs up as straight as possible, then reach up for your feet. [2] Slowly lower your left arm and left leg towards the ground, stopping just before you touch (this should take 4sec). At the same time, your right hand should be touching your right shin, but not holding on. [3] Slowly squeeze back to the top, focusing on pulling up through your toes (again this should take 4sec). [4] Next time, start by lowering your right arm and right leg. Alternate each time.

Jabs: orthodox (left)
20sec ON / 10sec REST

[1] Stand in orthodox position: left shoulder facing your 'target', feet hip-width apart, right fist next to your chin and left fist just in front of your face. [2] Extend your left arm out straight, knuckles aimed at your target. [3] As soon as your elbow straightens, quickly drag your elbow and fist back to the start, then fire it back out. [4] The rhythm is: jab-jab-rest-jab-jab-rest.

Repeat this exercise but for 20sec on and 60sec rest on the right-hand side.

→ DAY ONE: **PART TWO** →

Step forward lunge
20sec ON / 10sec REST

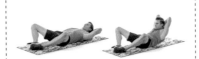

[1] Stand with your feet hip-width apart and your hands on your hips. Take a big step forward with your right foot. You should now be up on your back toes. [2] Lower your back knee towards the ground, stopping about 2.5 cm (1 inch) short. [3] Drive up hard from your right heel, pushing back to your start position.

Repeat this exercise with the left leg.

Monk crunches
40sec ON / 20sec REST

[1] Lie down on your back with your knees spread and the soles of your feet together. The closer you can pull your heels up towards your glutes, the better. [2] Reach across the back of your head and place each hand on your opposite shoulder. [3] Squeeze your rib cage towards your pelvis as hard as possible, lifting your shoulder blades off the ground while leaving your lower back on the ground. [4] Hold at the top of the movement for a second before slowly lowering yourself back down.

Jab–jab–cross: orthodox
20sec ON / 10sec REST

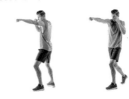

[1] Follow steps 1 to 3 of 'Jabs: orthodox' (above). [2] As your left arm is coming back from the second punch, throw your right arm out, aiming your right fist at the 'target'. As soon as your right elbow straightens, drag the right arm back until you are back in the start position. [3] The rhythm is: jab-jab-cross-rest-jab-jab-cross-rest.

Repeat this exercise but for 20sec on and 60sec rest on the right-hand side.

Pike squats
20sec ON / 10sec REST

[1] Stand with your feet together and your knees unlocked. Reach down and grab hold of your toes. [2] Rolling onto the balls of your feet, sit down until your butt is resting on the back of your calves. [3] Without letting go, drive your hips back up as high as you can, driving down through your heels at the same time. Don't let go of your toes until you have completed the full set.

Repeat this exercise.

Ankle taps
40sec ON / 20sec REST

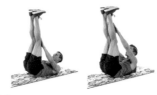

[1] Lie on your back with your legs straight up in the air and your hands resting on your knees. [2] Squeeze your rib cage towards your pelvis as hard as you can, sliding your hands up your shins until you reach your ankles. [3] Slowly lower yourself back down.

Jab–jab–cross–hook: orthodox
20sec ON / 10sec REST

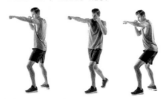

[1] Complete as for 'Jab-jab-cross: orthodox' (page 43), but this time as soon as your right elbow straightens, drag the right arm back and swing your left arm across your body at shoulder level, with your palm facing down. Imagine you are striking across the front of your target. [2] The rhythm is: jab-jab-cross-hook-rest-jab-jab-cross-hook-rest.

Repeat this exercise but for 20sec on and 60sec rest on the right-hand side.

DAY 2:
DAYS TO WOW: *41*

WORKING ON:
CHEST, BACK

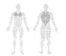

Repeat
3
Rounds

Stutter push-ups
20sec ON / 10sec REST

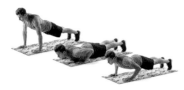

[1] Take up the military push-up position with your hands shoulder-width apart and your feet slightly apart. [2] Keeping your body locked tight, slowly lower your chest towards the floor. [3] Once your chest touches, push down hard through the heels of your palms, driving back up until your shoulders are at elbow level. [4] Lower yourself back down until your chest touches the floor again, then drive all the way back up to the start position.

Supine iron cross
20sec ON / 10sec REST

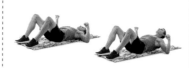

[1] Lie on your back with your knees bent at 90 degrees and your arms out to the sides at shoulder level and bent at 90 degrees. Make a fist with each hand and point your thumbs straight up towards the ceiling. [2] Keeping your body locked, push down as hard as you can through your elbows until your shoulders peel up off the ground. [3] When you can't get any higher, hold the position for a second, then slowly lower yourself down to the ground.

High knees
20sec ON / 10sec REST

[1] Start jogging on the spot, holding your hands out in front of you at waist level. [2] Pick up the intensity by pulling up through your knees until they are right up at waist level. Be careful not to lean back. Keep your stomach tight.

Repeat this exercise but for 20sec on and 60sec rest.

Wide-hand push-ups

20sec ON / 10sec REST

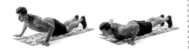

[1] Take up the standard push-up position, but have your hands out 2.5–5 cm (1–2 inches) wider than your shoulders and your fingers pointed out at 45 degrees. [2] Keeping your body locked tight, slowly lower your chest towards the floor. [3] Once your chest touches, push down hard through the heels of your palms, driving back up until your elbows are straight.

Fonzarelli push-ups

20sec ON / 10sec REST

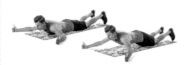

[1] Lie on your stomach with your arms stretched out at 45 degrees (your body should look like a 'Y'). [2] Make a fist with each hand and point your thumbs straight up towards the ceiling (like 'Fonzie'). [3] Keeping your body locked and your knees on the floor, push down as hard as you can through each fist, lifting your torso up off the ground. [4] When you can't get any higher, hold for a second, then slowly lower your torso back to the ground.

Boots to glutes

20sec ON / 10sec REST

[1] Start jogging on the spot. [2] Next, start pulling your heels up high, straight underneath you, as if trying to tap them on the spot where your butt meets your hamstrings.

> **Repeat this exercise but for 20sec on and 60sec rest.**

Elbows to hands

20sec ON / 10sec REST

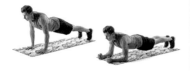

[1] Take up the standard push-up position, but have your feet hip-width apart. [2] Pick up your right hand and replace it with your right elbow. Pick up your left hand and replace it with your left elbow. You should now be in the plank position. [3] Pick up your right elbow and put your right hand back where it started, then pick up your left elbow and do the same thing with your left hand. You should now be back in the push-up position. [4] Next time, start by picking up your left hand. Alternate each time.

Prone crucifix raise

20sec ON / 10sec REST

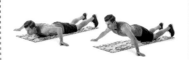

[1] Lie on your stomach with your arms out to the sides at shoulder level, and your elbows slightly bent. [2] Keeping your knees on the ground, and your body locked, push down hard through the heels of your palms, lifting your upper body up off the ground. [3] When you can't get any higher, hold for a second, then slowly lower your chest back down to the ground.

Fast feet

20sec ON / 10sec REST

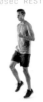

[1] Start by jogging on the spot. [2] Next, start taking tiny steps on the spot, sprinting as hard as you can and driving your arms hard to help keep up the pace.

> **Repeat this exercise but for 20sec on and 60sec rest.**

SORE MUSCLES MEAN PROGRESS. STAY FOCUSED, STAY ON COURSE.

DAY 3:
DAYS TO WOW: *40*

WORKING ON:
BICEPS, TRICEPS

Repeat
3
Rounds

→ DAY THREE: PART ONE →

Foot-resisted towel curl with supination

20sec ON / 10sec REST

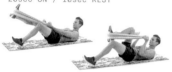

[1] Lie on your back with your preferred knee to your chest. [2] Hook a bath towel over your foot and grip both ends of the towel. [3] Push against the towel with your foot, extending your leg while resisting with your arms. [4] Once your arms are straight, bend your elbows and fold your arms as if trying to touch your forearms to your biceps. At the same time, rotate your palms so your thumbs point out to the sides. Keep tension on the towel with your foot but don't stop your arms folding.

Prayer push-ups

20sec ON / 10sec REST

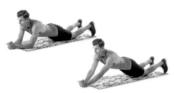

[1] Take up the plank position, with your feet together and your elbows directly under your shoulders. [2] Rest your knees on the ground and keep your body locked. Lace your fingers together as if you are praying. [3] Push down as hard as you can with your hands, straightening your elbows and lifting your torso up off the ground. [4] When you can't get any higher, hold for a second, then slowly lower yourself back to the start position.

Pseudo-skipping: jumps

20sec ON / 10sec REST

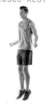

[1] Hold your hands beside you as if you're holding a skipping rope. [2] Start to rotate your hands as if you're swinging a rope. [3] Each time your hands hit the lowest point of the circle, push off your toes and bounce up off the ground as if you're jumping over the rope. Be sure to keep time with your hands.

> **Repeat this exercise but for 20sec on and 60sec rest.**

→ DAY THREE: PART TWO →

Bicep push-ups

20sec ON / 10sec REST

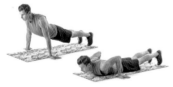

[1] Take up the standard push-up position, then turn your hands all the way out until your fingers are pointing down towards your feet. [2] Keeping your body locked tight, slowly lower your chest towards the floor. Your elbows should be scraping against your ribs. [3] Once your chest touches, push down hard through the heels of your palms, driving back up until your elbows are straight.

Tiger push-ups

20sec ON / 10sec REST

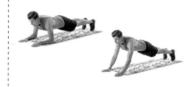

[1] Start in the plank position, with your feet slightly apart and your elbows directly under your shoulders. [2] Keeping your body locked tight, push down hard through the heels of your palms, straightening your elbows until they lift up off the ground. [3] Slowly bend your elbows and gently lower yourself back down.

> **NOTE: If you are unable to do this exercise on your toes, place your knees on the ground, keep your body locked and keep going.**

Pseudo-skipping: double steps

20sec ON / 10sec REST

[1] Start by balancing on your left foot, and start to rotate your hands as if swinging a rope. [2] When your hands hit the lowest point of the circle, push off your toes and bounce up off your left foot. As your hands come around again, bounce on your left foot a second time. [3] The next time, bounce on your right foot for two cycles before switching back to your left.

> **Repeat this exercise but for 20sec on and 60sec rest.**

Foot-resisted towel rows

20sec ON / 10sec REST

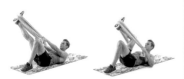

[1] Sit with your legs straight out in front of you, with your preferred knee to your chest. [2] Hook a bath towel over your foot and grip both ends of the towel. [3] Push against the towel with your foot, extending your leg while resisting with your arms. [4] Once your arms are straight, pull your elbows straight back past your ribs. At the same time, keep tension on the towel with your foot. The trick to this exercise is to apply as much pressure through your foot as you can without stopping your arms from moving.

Kneeling tricep extension

20sec ON / 10sec REST

[1] Push a chair or stool up against something to stop it from moving. Kneel down in front of it so that your outstretched fingers are 5 cm (2 inches) from the edge. [2] Squeezing your glutes and keeping your body locked, lean forward until your hands rest on the edge of the chair. [3] Bend your elbows, pointing them down towards the ground, and lower yourself down until your chin touches the edge of the chair. [4] Push down hard through your palms, straightening your elbows and driving back up to the start position.

Pseudo-skipping: hops

20sec ON / 10sec REST

[1] Start by balancing on your left foot, and start to rotate your hands as if swinging a rope. [2] Each time your hands hit the lowest point of the circle, push off your toes and hop up off the ground as if you're jumping over the rope, landing back on your left foot each time. Be sure to keep time with your hands.

> **Repeat this exercise but on the right side for 20sec on and 60sec rest.**

DAY 4:
DAYS TO WOW: 39

WORKING ON:
SHOULDERS, CORE

Repeat 3 Rounds

Foot-resisted towel upright rows

20sec ON / 10sec REST

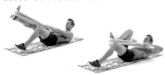

[1] Lie on your back, with your preferred knee to your chest. [2] Hook a bath towel over your foot and grip both ends of the towel. [3] Push against the towel with your foot, extending your leg while resisting with your arms. [4] Once your arms are straight, bend your elbows out to the sides, lifting them as high as possible. At the same time, keep tension on the towel with your foot. The trick is to apply as much pressure through your foot as you can without stopping your arms from moving.

Plank hold with Superman reach

40sec ON / 20sec REST

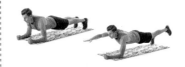

[1] Take up the plank position, resting on your elbows and toes. Your feet should be shoulder-width apart. [2] Lift up your left leg and point your toe. At the same time, lift up your right arm and reach it straight out in front of you as if you're flying like Superman. [3] Slowly lower your leg and arm down so you are back in the plank position, then repeat the process using your right leg and left arm.

Step back lunge to knee drive

20sec ON / 10sec REST

[1] Stand with your feet hip-width apart. Take a big step backwards with your right foot so you are resting on the tips of your toes. [2] Lower your right knee straight down, stopping 2.5 cm (1 inch) off the ground. [3] Drive down through your left heel and punch your right knee up as if kneeing someone in the belly. [4] Swing your right leg back again and drop into another lunge.

> **Repeat this exercise but on the left side for 20sec on and 60sec rest.**

Dive bombers

20sec ON / 10sec REST

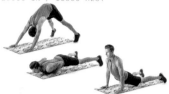

[1] Take up the standard push-up position, but have your feet shoulder-width apart and hips as high as possible. [2] Bend your elbows and lower yourself as if you are going to touch your forehead to the ground between your hands. Before it touches, slide your body forward as if you are going to touch your nose, then chin, chest and hips in the same spot. [3] Next, arch your back and straighten your elbows. [4] Reverse the action, bending your elbows and lowering your chest back to the ground.

Leg raises

40sec ON / 20sec REST

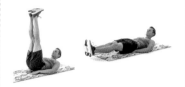

[1] Lie on your back with your hands under your butt. [2] Bend your knees and lift your legs up until they are pointing straight up in the air. [3] Squeeze your rib cage towards your hips, tightening your abs. [4] Slowly lower your legs down towards the ground, keeping them as straight as possible. Before they touch the ground, stop and hold for a second. [5] Pulling through your toes, slowly bring your legs back up so they are pointing straight up in the air.

Lateral jumps

20sec ON / 10sec REST

[1] Start with your feet hip-width apart and your arms by your sides. [2] Lower yourself down into a half-squat, reaching forward with your arms as you do. [3] Drive up, swing your arms back past your hips and leap as far to your left as you can. [4] Land with soft knees, dropping straight back down into a half-squat. [5] This time when you drive back up, leap as far to your right as you can.

> **Repeat this exercise but for 20sec on and 60sec rest.**

Prone upper-body snow angels

20sec ON / 10sec REST

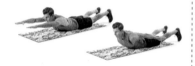

[1] Lie on your stomach with your arms stretched out above your head. [2] Lift your arms and chest off the ground, keeping your toes in contact with the ground. [3] Keeping your arms off the ground, swing them wide around your body until your hands touch your hips. [4] Keep your arms and chest up as you swing your arms back above your head.

Flutter kicks

40sec ON / 20sec REST

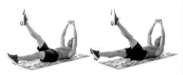

[1] Lie on your back and bring your knees up to your chest. [2] Reach your arms up towards the ceiling, squeezing your rib cage towards your pelvis and curling your shoulder blades off the ground. [3] Keeping your stomach tight, extend your legs and start kicking as if you were doing backstroke. Keep your knees straight. When you reach the end of the set, bend your knees before you lower your feet to the ground.

High heel taps

20sec ON / 10sec REST

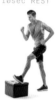

[1] Stand in front of a step or something similar that is about 20 cm (8 inches) high. [2] Rest the back of your right heel on the edge of the step, with your weight on your left leg. [3] Jump up and switch legs so that you are now standing on your right leg and the back of your left heel is resting on the step.

> **Repeat this exercise but for 20sec on and 60sec rest.**

DON'T LET ANYTHING STAND BETWEEN YOU AND YOUR GOALS. YOU'RE HALFWAY THERE.

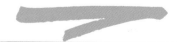

DAY 1:
DAYS TO WOW: *28*

WORKING ON:
LEGS, GLUTES, ABS

→ DAY ONE: PART ONE →

Goblet squats
50sec ON / 10sec REST

[1] Stand with your feet hip-width apart. Lace your fingers together at chin height with your elbows pointing straight down. [2] Keeping your weight on your heels, sit down as deep as possible, until your elbows are between your knees. [3] Drive down hard through your heels and stand back up straight.

Jackknives
50sec ON / 10sec REST

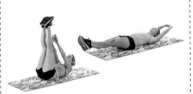

[1] Lie on your back, bend your knees and bring your legs up as straight as possible, then reach up for your ankles. [2] From here, slowly lower your hands and feet towards the ground, stopping just before you touch (this should take 4sec). [3] Slowly squeeze back to the top, focusing on pulling up through your toes (again this should take 4sec).

Upper-body jumping jacks
30sec ON / 15sec REST

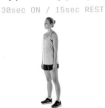 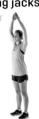

[1] Stand with your feet slightly apart, your knees unlocked and your arms by your sides. [2] Keeping your arms straight, swing them out to the sides and straight up above your head until your hands touch. [3] Swing your arms back down until your palms slap the outside of your thighs.

> **Repeat this exercise but for 30sec on and 30sec rest.**

→ DAY ONE: PART TWO →

Bulgarian split squat
30sec ON / 15sec REST

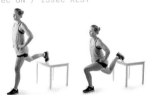

[1] Stand one stride in front of a chair or low table, then lift up your right foot, reach back and put your toes on the chair. [2] With your hands resting on your hips, bend your left knee and lower yourself down, pushing your right knee back towards the chair. [3] Now press down through your left heel and drive up until your left knee is straight.

> **Repeat this exercise with the right leg.**

Supine window washers
50sec ON / 10sec REST

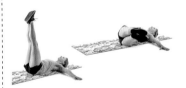

[1] Lie on your back with your arms stretched out to the sides, palms down. [2] Bend your knees and bring your legs up as straight as possible. [3] Slowly lower your legs down to the left, stopping just short of the floor, then slowly bring your legs back up until they are directly over your hips. [4] Repeat, lowering your legs down to the right.

Upper-body cross countries
30sec ON / 15sec REST

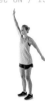 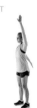

[1] Stand with your feet slightly apart and your knees unlocked. [2] Swing your right arm forward as high as possible as you swing your left arm back as far as possible. [3] Now swing your arms through as fast as possible until your left arm is above your head to the front, and your right arm is stretched back behind you.

> **Repeat this exercise but for 30sec on and 30sec rest.**

Supine hamstring curl
30sec ON / 15sec REST

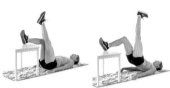

[1] Lie on your back directly in front of a chair or low table with your right knee bent and your right heel on the chair. Straighten your left leg. [2] Push down as hard as you can through your right heel, squeezing your glutes. Your hips will start to rise up off the floor. [3] Hold at the top of the movement for a two-count, then slowly lower your hips back down.

Repeat this exercise with the left leg.

Low-profile sit-ups
50sec ON / 10sec REST

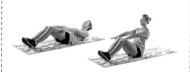

[1] Lie on your back with your knees bent at 90 degrees and your hands beside your thighs. [2] Squeeze your rib cage towards your pelvis and reach forward until your thumbs are alongside your kneecaps. [3] Slowly lower your shoulders back down towards the floor.

Upper-body SEAL jacks
30sec ON / 15sec REST

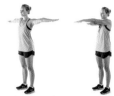

[1] Stand with your feet hip-width apart and your arms stretched straight out to the sides, palms down, at shoulder level. [2] Keeping your arms at shoulder level, swing them forward until your elbows cross in front of you. [3] Next, again keeping your arms up at shoulder level, swing them back as far as possible.

Repeat this exercise but for 30sec on and 30sec rest.

DAY 2:
DAYS TO WOW: *27*

WORKING ON:
CHEST, BACK

Repeat 3 Rounds

Deep push-ups
30sec ON / 15sec REST

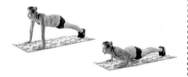

[1] Take up the military push-up position with your hands shoulder-width apart and your feet together. [2] Keeping your body locked tight, slowly lower your chest towards the floor. [3] Once your chest touches the floor, push down hard through the heels of your palms, driving back up until your elbows are straight.

Supine elbow push-ups
30sec ON / 15sec REST

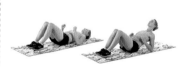

[1] Lie on your back with your knees and elbows bent at 90 degrees and your arms at a 45-degree angle from your body. [2] Press down through your elbows as hard as you can, lifting your shoulder blades up off the ground. [3] Slowly lower yourself back down to the floor.

Squat jumps
30sec ON / 15sec REST

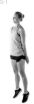

[1] Stand with your feet hip-width apart. [2] Sit down into a deep squat with your weight on your heels and your arms stretched out in front of you. [3] Drive down through your heels and leap up tall. [4] Land with bent knees and drop straight down into the next squat.

Repeat this exercise but for 30sec on and 30sec rest.

Decline push-ups

30sec ON / 15sec REST

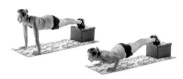

[1] Take up the standard push-up position, with your toes up on a low stool or similar. [2] Keeping your body locked, lower your chest towards the ground. [3] Push down hard through the heels of your palms and drive back up until your elbows are straight.

NOTE: To reduce the intensity, rest your knees on the stool instead of your toes.

Downward dog to cobra

30sec ON / 15sec REST

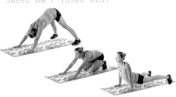

[1] Take up the standard push-up position. Move your feet shoulder-width apart, push your hips up high and walk your hands back towards your feet until you're looking straight back through your knees. [2] Now, bend your knees, lowering them until they are about 2.5 cm (1 inch) from the floor. [3] Push your hips forward and down until they are 2.5 cm (1 inch) from the floor. Your elbows should be straight, and your chest up tall. [4] Reverse the movement until you are back in the original downward dog position.

Switch lunges

30sec ON / 15sec REST

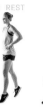

[1] Stand with your feet hip-width apart and your hands on your hips. Take a big step forward with your right foot. You should now be up on your back toes. [2] Lower your back knee down towards the ground, then drive up and switch your legs so that your left leg is now in front. [3] Lower your back knee down towards the ground, then drive up and switch your legs again.

Repeat this exercise but for 30sec on and 30sec rest.

Close-grip push-ups

30sec ON / 15sec REST

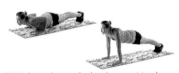

[1] Take up the standard push-up position, but place your hands down a little closer to your hips than usual. [2] As you lower yourself down towards the ground, leading with your chest, your elbows should slide tightly past your rib cage. [3] Once your chest touches the ground, push down hard through the heels of your palms and drive back up until your elbows are straight.

Doorframe rows

30sec ON / 15sec REST

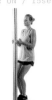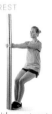

[1] Stand in a doorway with your toes touching the doorframe and your knees slightly bent, gripping the doorframe with both hands. [2] Keeping your heels on the ground, lock your body, extend your arms and lean back. [3] Now, keeping your body locked straight, drag your elbows back past your ribs, pulling yourself towards the doorframe. [4] When your knees are almost touching the doorframe, pause for a second before extending your arms and slowly lowering yourself backwards again.

Switch squats

30sec ON / 15sec REST

[1] Stand with your feet 5 cm (2 inches) apart, toes straight ahead. [2] Sit into a deep squat with your weight on your heels and your arms out in front. [3] Drive down through your heels and leap up tall, landing with your heels wide and your toes at 45 degrees. [4] Sit into a sumo squat, keeping your knees in line with your toes, then leap up and land in the original position.

Repeat this exercise but for 30sec on and 30sec rest.

KEEP YOUR EYES ON THE PRIZE! THAT FINISH LINE IS GETTING CLOSER.

DAY 3:

DAYS TO WOW: *26*

WORKING ON:

BICEPS, TRICEPS

→ DAY THREE: PART ONE →

Doorframe bicep curls

30sec ON / 15sec REST

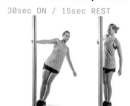

[1] Stand in a doorway, facing the doorframe. Lift your right arm up to shoulder level and clasp the edge of the doorframe with your fingertips. [2] Keeping your elbow at shoulder level, lock your body and bend your elbow, pulling your right shoulder towards the doorframe. [3] Slowly straighten your arm and push yourself back to the start position.

Repeat this exercise on the left side.

Tricep dips

30sec ON / 15sec REST

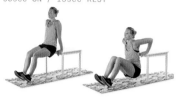

[1] Push a chair or low table up against something to stop it from moving. Sit on the edge of the chair with your palms flat and your thumbs under the edge of your butt. [2] Take your weight onto your hands, sliding your hips forward off the edge of the chair. [3] Bend your elbows and lower your butt towards the floor, keeping your back as close to the chair as possible. [4] When you can't get any lower, push down hard through your hands and drive back up until your elbows are straight.

Mountain climbers

30sec ON / 15sec REST

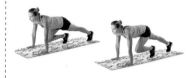

[1] Take up the standard push-up position. Keeping your body locked, bring your right knee up towards your chest and rest your toe on the floor. [2] Keeping tight through your mid-section, push off your right foot and switch legs so that your left knee is pulled up towards your chest. [3] Push off your left foot and switch legs again.

Repeat this exercise but for 30sec on and 30sec rest.

→ DAY THREE: PART TWO →

Seated towel curls

30sec ON / 15sec REST

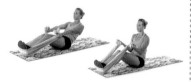

[1] Sit on the ground with your knees bent at 90 degrees. [2] Hook a bath towel over your feet and grip both ends of the towel. [3] With your palms facing up, slowly straighten your arms, lowering your shoulders towards the floor. [4] Now, bend your elbows as if you are trying to touch your knuckles to your collarbone. Try to push your weight back through your shoulders in order to create as much resistance as possible.

Badger push-ups

30sec ON / 15sec REST

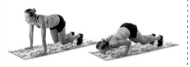

[1] Take up the table-top position, with your hands directly under your shoulders and knees directly under your hips. Push down into the floor with your toes so that your knees are 2.5 cm (1 inch) off the ground. [2] Sit back on your haunches, with your butt resting on your calves. [3] Bend your elbows and aim to touch your chin on the ground between your fingertips. [4] Leading with your hips, push down hard through your palms and drive back until your butt is resting on your calves again.

Frogs

30sec ON / 15sec REST

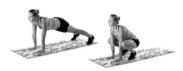

[1] Take up the standard push-up position. Drive down hard through your toes and pull your knees up either side of your elbows until you are in the frog position. [2] Shift your weight back over your hands and kick back out into the push-up position again.

Repeat this exercise but for 30sec on and 30sec rest.

Leg-resisted hammer curls
30sec ON / 15sec REST

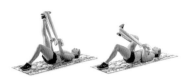

[1] Lie on your back, hook a bath towel over your right foot and grip both ends of the towel. [2] Push your foot up while resisting with your arms. [3] Once your arms are straight, bend your elbows and fold your arms as if you are trying to touch your thumbs to your shoulders. At the same time, keep tension on the towel with your foot and don't let your arms fold.

Repeat this exercise on the left side.

Diamond push-ups
30sec ON / 15sec REST

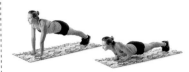

[1] Take up the standard push-up position, but bring your hands together under your chest, creating a diamond shape with your index fingers and thumbs. Your hands need to be a little lower than the standard push-up position. [2] Bend your elbows and lower yourself down until your chest touches the back of your hands. [3] Now, keeping your body locked, push down hard through your palms and drive back up until your elbows are straight.

Squat thrust
30sec ON / 15sec REST

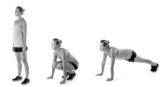

[1] Stand up straight with your feet hip-width apart. [2] Drop down until your butt is resting on the back of your calves, with your hands on the floor. [3] Shift your weight over your hands and kick out into a push-up position. [4] Jump back into the crouch position, with your knees between your elbows. [5] Drive down through your heels and stand up tall.

Repeat this exercise for 30sec on and 30sec rest.

DAY 4:
DAYS TO WOW: 25

WORKING ON:
SHOULDERS, ABS

Repeat 3 Rounds

Shoulder push-ups
30sec ON / 15sec REST

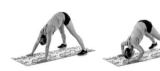

[1] Take up the standard push-up position. Move your feet out to shoulder width, push your hips up high and walk your hands back towards your feet until you're looking straight back through your knees. Turn your fingers in slightly. [2] Slowly bend your elbows and lower yourself down, aiming to touch the top of your head gently on the ground between your hands. [3] Push down hard through your palms and drive back up until your elbows are straight.

Stutter sit-ups
50sec ON / 10sec REST

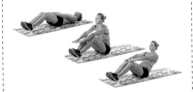

[1] Start in the standard military sit-up position, with your knees bent at 90 degrees and your hands resting on your thighs. [2] Squeeze your rib cage towards your pelvis, sliding your hands along your thighs until your elbows are resting on your knees. [3] Slowly lower yourself back until your palms are resting on your knees, but your back is still off the ground. [4] Squeeze back up until your elbows are back on your knees. [5] Lower back down to the start position.

Speed skaters
30sec ON / 15sec REST

[1] Stand with your feet hip-width apart. [2] Leap as wide to the left as possible, landing on your left foot and swinging your right leg behind your left. [3] Swing your right leg back out to the right, leaping as wide as possible and landing on your right foot, swinging your left leg behind your right leg.

Repeat this exercise but for 30sec on and 30sec rest.

Hindu push-ups

30sec ON / 15sec REST

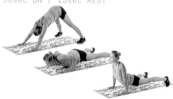

[1] Take up the standard push-up position, but have your feet shoulder-width apart and your hips as high in the air as possible. [2] Bend your elbows and lower yourself as if you are going to touch your forehead to the ground between your hands. Before it touches, slide your body forward as if you are going to touch your nose, then chin, chest and hips in the same spot. [3] Once your hips are in line with your hands, arch your back and straighten your elbows. [4] Lift your hips as high as possible and push into the start position.

Push-up position hold

50sec ON / 10sec REST

[1] Take up the standard military push-up position. [2] Hold this position for the prescribed time, ensuring you keep a straight line between your shoulders, hips and ankles.

NOTE: Be careful not to drop or lift your hips.

High jumps

30sec ON / 15sec REST

[1] Stand with your feet hip-width apart. [2] Sit into a half-squat with your arms in front of you. [3] Swing your arms back past your hips, leaping up as high as possible. At the same time, draw your knees up towards your chest until you are in a tuck position in midair. [4] Land with bent knees and drop straight down into the next half-squat.

Repeat this exercise but for 30sec on and 30sec rest.

Cross-body ankle taps

30sec ON / 15sec REST

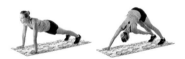

[1] Take up the standard push-up position, with your feet shoulder-width apart. [2] Drive your hips upwards, then pick up your left hand and reach through to tap your right ankle. [3] Lower yourself back down to a dead-straight push-up position. [4] Drive your hips back up, then pick up your right hand and reach through to tap your left ankle. [5] Return to a dead-straight push-up position.

Overhead sit-ups

50sec ON / 10sec REST

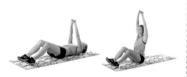

[1] Start in the standard military sit-up position, with your knees bent at 90 degrees and your arms straight up as if you are reaching for the ceiling. [2] Squeeze your rib cage towards your hips and drive up into a seated position. Your arms should still be stretched up towards the sky. [3] Slowly lower yourself back down to the start position.

Toe taps

30sec ON / 15sec REST

[1] Stand in front of a step or something similar that is about 20 cm (8 inches) high. [2] Rest the bottom of your right toes on the edge of the step, with your weight on your left leg. [3] Jump up and switch legs so that you are standing on your right leg, with your left toes resting on the step.

Repeat this exercise but for 30sec on and 30sec rest.

EMBRACE THE UNCOMFORTABLE AND YOU WILL GO FURTHER THAN YOU CAN IMAGINE.

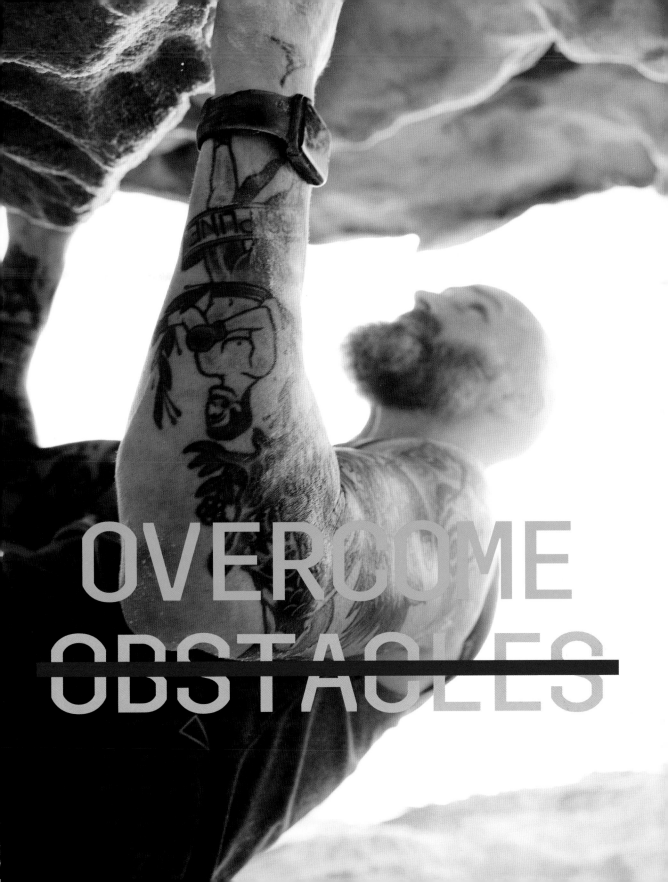

OVERCOME
~~OBSTACLES~~

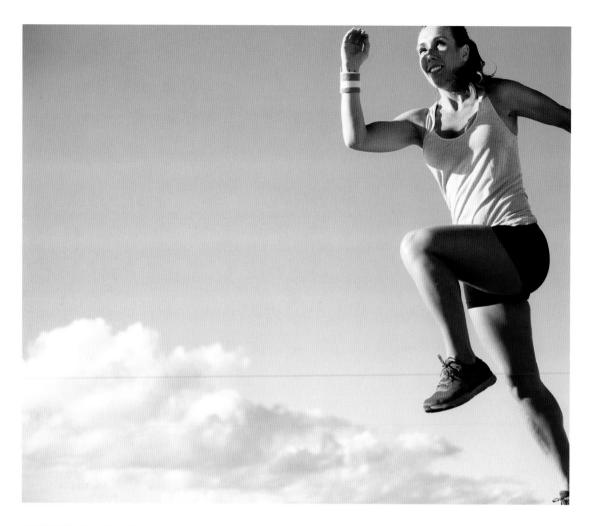

The home straight

By now, you must be on a results-inspired high. You're leaner, stronger, more athletic and, most importantly, you feel great. This is the time to harness all that positive energy and to make every rep of every set of the next 2 weeks count.

Once again, we are returning to exercises that you know well, so there's no excuse for poor form, or a lack of intensity. Think about how far you've come over the past 6 weeks, and visualise exactly where you want to be in 2 weeks' time.

DAY 1:
DAYS TO WOW: *14*

WORKING ON:
LEGS, GLUTES, ABS

→ DAY ONE: PART ONE →

Stutter squats
30sec ON / 15sec REST

[1] Stand with your feet hip-width apart, hands by your sides. [2] Leading with your glutes, sit into a deep squat, reaching forward with your arms in order to stay balanced. Your goal is to get your butt to the back of your calves (or as close as possible). [3] Come halfway up, until your thighs are parallel to the ground. [4] Lower back down again, then drive all the way back up to a standing position.

Pocket knives
50sec ON / 10sec REST

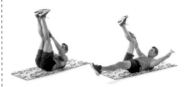

[1] Lie on your back, bend your knees and bring your legs up as straight as possible, then reach up for your feet. [2] Slowly lower your left arm and left leg towards the ground, stopping just before you touch (this should take 4sec). At the same time, your right hand should be touching your right shin, but not holding on. [3] Slowly squeeze back to the top, focusing on pulling up through your toes (again this should take 4sec). [4] Next time, start by lowering your right arm and right leg. Alternate each time.

Jabs: orthodox (left)
30sec ON / 15sec REST

[1] Stand in orthodox position: left shoulder facing your 'target', feet hip-width apart, right fist next to your chin and left fist just in front of your face. [2] Extend your left arm out straight, knuckles aimed at your target. [3] As soon as your elbow straightens, quickly drag your elbow and fist back to the start, then fire it back out. [4] The rhythm is: jab-jab-rest-jab-jab-rest.

Repeat this exercise but for 30sec on and 30sec rest on the right-hand side.

→ DAY ONE: PART TWO →

Step forward lunge
30sec ON / 15sec REST

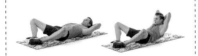

[1] Stand with your feet hip-width apart and your hands on your hips. Take a big step forward with your right foot. You should now be up on your back toes. [2] Lower your back knee towards the ground, stopping about 2.5 cm (1 inch) short. [3] Drive up hard from your right heel, pushing back to your start position.

Repeat this exercise with the left leg.

Monk crunches
50sec ON / 10sec REST

[1] Lie down on your back with your knees spread and the soles of your feet together. The closer you can pull your heels up towards your glutes, the better. [2] Reach across the back of your head and place each hand on your opposite shoulder. [3] Squeeze your rib cage towards your pelvis as hard as possible, lifting your shoulder blades off the ground while leaving your lower back on the ground. [4] Hold at the top of the movement for a second before slowly lowering yourself back down.

Jab–jab–cross: orthodox
30sec ON / 15sec REST

[1] Follow steps 1 to 3 of 'Jabs: orthodox' (above). [2] As your left arm is coming back from the second punch, throw your right arm out, aiming your right fist at the 'target'. As soon as your right elbow straightens, drag the right arm back until you are back in the start position. [3] The rhythm is: jab-jab-cross-rest-jab-jab-cross-rest.

Repeat this exercise but for 30sec on and 30sec rest on the right-hand side.

59

Pike squats
30sec ON / 15sec REST

[1] Stand with your feet together and your knees unlocked. Reach down and grab hold of your toes. [2] Rolling onto the balls of your feet, sit down until your butt is resting on the back of your calves. [3] Without letting go, drive your hips back up as high as you can, driving down through your heels at the same time. Don't let go of your toes until you have completed the full set.

Repeat this exercise.

Ankle taps
50sec ON / 10sec REST

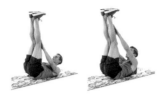

[1] Lie on your back with your legs straight up in the air and your hands resting on your knees. [2] Squeeze your rib cage towards your pelvis as hard as you can, sliding your hands up your shins until you reach your ankles. [3] Slowly lower yourself back down.

Jab–jab–cross–hook: orthodox
30sec ON / 15sec REST

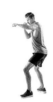

[1] Complete as for 'Jab-jab-cross: orthodox' (page 59), but this time as soon as your right elbow straightens, drag the right arm back and swing your left arm across your body at shoulder level, with your palm facing down. Imagine you are striking across the front of your target. [2] The rhythm is: jab-jab-cross-hook-rest-jab-jab-cross-hook-rest.

Repeat this exercise but for 30sec on and 30sec rest on the right-hand side.

DAY 2:
DAYS TO WOW: *13*

WORKING ON:
CHEST, BACK

Repeat
3
Rounds

Stutter push-ups
30sec ON / 15sec REST

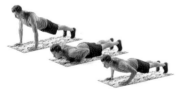

[1] Take up the military push-up position with your hands shoulder-width apart and your feet slightly apart. [2] Keeping your body locked tight, slowly lower your chest towards the floor. [3] Once your chest touches, push down hard through the heels of your palms, driving back up until your shoulders are at elbow level. [4] Lower yourself back down until your chest touches the floor again, then drive all the way back up to the start position.

Supine iron cross
30sec ON / 15sec REST

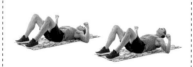

[1] Lie on your back with your knees bent at 90 degrees and your arms out to the sides at shoulder level and bent at 90 degrees. Make a fist with each hand and point your thumbs straight up towards the ceiling. [2] Keeping your body locked, push down as hard as you can through your elbows until your shoulders peel up off the ground. [3] When you can't get any higher, hold the position for a second, then slowly lower yourself down to the ground.

High knees
30sec ON / 15sec REST

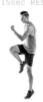

[1] Start jogging on the spot, holding your hands out in front of you at waist level. [2] Pick up the intensity by pulling up through your knees until they are right up at waist level. Be careful not to lean back. Keep your stomach tight.

Repeat this exercise but for 30sec on and 30sec rest.

Wide-hand push-ups

30sec ON / 15sec REST

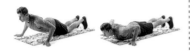

[1] Take up the standard push-up position, but have your hands out 2.5-5 cm (1-2 inches) wider than your shoulders and your fingers pointed out at 45 degrees. [2] Keeping your body locked tight, slowly lower your chest towards the floor. [3] Once your chest touches, push down hard through the heels of your palms, driving back up until your elbows are straight.

Fonzarelli push-ups

30sec ON / 15sec REST

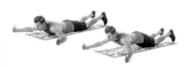

[1] Lie on your stomach with your arms stretched out at 45 degrees (your body should look like a 'Y'). [2] Make a fist with each hand and point your thumbs straight up towards the ceiling (like 'Fonzie'). [3] Keeping your body locked and your knees on the floor, push down as hard as you can through each fist, lifting your torso up off the ground. [4] When you can't get any higher, hold for a second, then slowly lower your torso back to the ground.

Boots to glutes

30sec ON / 15sec REST

[1] Start jogging on the spot. [2] Next, start pulling your heels up high, straight underneath you, as if trying to tap them on the spot where your butt meets your hamstrings.

Repeat this exercise but for 30sec on and 30sec rest.

Elbows to hands

30sec ON / 15sec REST

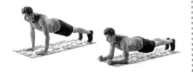

[1] Take up the standard push-up position, but have your feet hip-width apart. [2] Pick up your right hand and replace it with your right elbow. Pick up your left hand and replace it with your left elbow. You should now be in the plank position. [3] Pick up your right elbow and put your right hand back where it started, then pick up your left elbow and do the same thing with your left hand. You should now be back in the push-up position. [4] Next time, start by picking up your left hand. Alternate each time.

Prone crucifix raise

30sec ON / 15sec REST

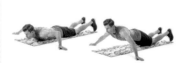

[1] Lie on your stomach with your arms out to the sides at shoulder level, and your elbows slightly bent. [2] Keeping your knees on the ground, and your body locked, push down hard through the heels of your palms, lifting your upper body up off the ground. [3] When you can't get any higher, hold for a second, then slowly lower your chest back down to the ground.

Fast feet

30sec ON / 15sec REST

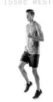

[1] Start by jogging on the spot. [2] Next, start taking tiny steps on the spot, sprinting as hard as you can and driving your arms hard to help keep up the pace.

Repeat this exercise but for 30sec on and 30sec rest.

HERE'S TO 7 WEEKS OF GRIT, DISCIPLINE AND NO EXCUSES. HERE'S TO CRUSHING IT.

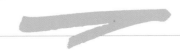

DAY 3:
DAYS TO WOW: *12*

WORKING ON:
BICEPS, TRICEPS

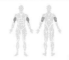

Repeat
3
Rounds

→ DAY THREE: PART ONE →

Foot-resisted towel curl with supination

30sec ON / 15sec REST

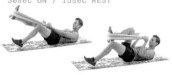

[1] Lie on your back with your preferred knee to your chest. [2] Hook a bath towel over your foot and grip both ends of the towel. [3] Push against the towel with your foot, extending your leg while resisting with your arms. [4] Once your arms are straight, bend your elbows and fold your arms as if trying to touch your forearms to your biceps. At the same time, rotate your palms so your thumbs point out to the sides. Keep tension on the towel with your foot but don't stop your arms folding.

Prayer push-ups

30sec ON / 15sec REST

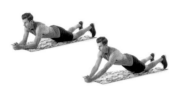

[1] Take up the plank position, with your feet together and your elbows directly under your shoulders. [2] Rest your knees on the ground and keep your body locked. Lace your fingers together as if you are praying. [3] Push down as hard as you can with your hands, straightening your elbows and lifting your torso up off the ground. [4] When you can't get any higher, hold for a second, then slowly lower yourself back to the start position.

Pseudo-skipping: jumps

30sec ON / 15sec REST

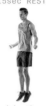

[1] Hold your hands beside you as if you're holding a skipping rope. [2] Start to rotate your hands as if you're swinging a rope. [3] Each time your hands hit the lowest point of the circle, push off your toes and bounce up off the ground as if you're jumping over the rope. Be sure to keep time with your hands.

Repeat this exercise but for 30sec on and 30sec rest.

→ DAY THREE: PART TWO →

Bicep push-ups

30sec ON / 15sec REST

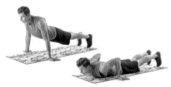

[1] Take up the standard push-up position, then turn your hands all the way out until your fingers are pointing down towards your feet. [2] Keeping your body locked tight, slowly lower your chest towards the floor. Your elbows should be scraping against your ribs. [3] Once your chest touches, push down hard through the heels of your palms, driving back up until your elbows are straight.

Tiger push-ups

30sec ON / 15sec REST

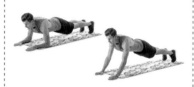

[1] Start in the plank position, with your feet slightly apart and your elbows directly under your shoulders. [2] Keeping your body locked tight, push down hard through the heels of your palms, straightening your elbows until they lift up off the ground. [3] Slowly bend your elbows and gently lower yourself back down.

NOTE: If you are unable to do this exercise on your toes, place your knees on the ground, keep your body locked and keep going.

Pseudo-skipping: double steps

30sec ON / 15sec REST

[1] Start by balancing on your left foot, and start to rotate your hands as if swinging a rope. [2] When your hands hit the lowest point of the circle, push off your toes and bounce up off your left foot. As your hands come around again, bounce on your left foot a second time. [3] The next time, bounce on your right foot for two cycles before switching back to your left.

Repeat this exercise but for 30sec on and 30sec rest.

Foot-resisted towel rows

30sec ON / 15sec REST

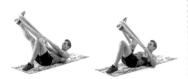

[1] Sit with your legs straight out in front of you, with your preferred knee to your chest. [2] Hook a bath towel over your foot and grip both ends of the towel. [3] Push against the towel with your foot, extending your leg while resisting with your arms. [4] Once your arms are straight, pull your elbows straight back past your ribs. At the same time, keep tension on the towel with your foot. The trick to this exercise is to apply as much pressure through your foot as you can without stopping your arms from moving.

Kneeling tricep extension

30sec ON / 15sec REST

[1] Push a chair or stool up against something to stop it from moving. Kneel down in front of it so that your outstretched fingers are 5 cm (2 inches) from the edge. [2] Squeezing your glutes and keeping your body locked, lean forward until your hands rest on the edge of the chair. [3] Bend your elbows, pointing them down towards the ground, and lower yourself down until your chin touches the edge of the chair. [4] Push down hard through your palms, straightening your elbows and driving back up to the start position.

Pseudo-skipping: hops

30sec ON / 15sec REST

[1] Start by balancing on your left foot, and start to rotate your hands as if swinging a rope. [2] Each time your hands hit the lowest point of the circle, push off your toes and hop up off the ground as if you're jumping over the rope, landing back on your left foot each time. Be sure to keep time with your hands.

Repeat this exercise but on the right side for 30sec on and 30sec rest.

DAY 4:
DAYS TO WOW: //

WORKING ON:
SHOULDERS, CORE

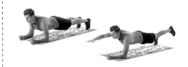

Repeat 3 Rounds

Foot-resisted towel upright rows

30sec ON / 15sec REST

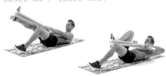

[1] Lie on your back, with your preferred knee to your chest. [2] Hook a bath towel over your foot and grip both ends of the towel. [3] Push against the towel with your foot, extending your leg while resisting with your arms. [4] Once your arms are straight, bend your elbows out to the sides, lifting them as high as possible. At the same time, keep tension on the towel with your foot. The trick is to apply as much pressure through your foot as you can without stopping your arms from moving.

Plank hold with Superman reach

50sec ON / 10sec REST

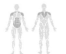

[1] Take up the plank position, resting on your elbows and toes. Your feet should be shoulder-width apart. [2] Lift up your left leg and point your toe. At the same time, lift up your right arm and reach it straight out in front of you as if you're flying like Superman. [3] Slowly lower your leg and arm down so you are back in the plank position, then repeat the process using your right leg and left arm.

Step back lunge to knee drive

30sec ON / 15sec REST

[1] Stand with your feet hip-width apart. Take a big step backwards with your right foot so you are resting on the tips of your toes. [2] Lower your right knee straight down, stopping 2.5 cm (1 inch) off the ground. [3] Drive down through your left heel and punch your right knee up as if kneeing someone in the belly. [4] Swing your right leg back again and drop into another lunge.

Repeat this exercise but on the left side for 30sec on and 30sec rest.

Dive bombers
30sec ON / 15sec REST

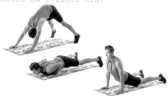

[1] Take up the standard push-up position, but have your feet shoulder-width apart and hips as high as possible. [2] Bend your elbows and lower yourself as if you are going to touch your forehead to the ground between your hands. Before it touches, slide your body forward as if you are going to touch your nose, then chin, chest and hips in the same spot. [3] Next, arch your back and straighten your elbows. [4] Reverse the action, bending your elbows and lowering your chest back to the ground.

Leg raises
50sec ON / 10sec REST

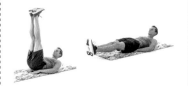

[1] Lie on your back with your hands under your butt. [2] Bend your knees and lift your legs up until they are pointing straight up in the air. [3] Squeeze your rib cage towards your hips, tightening your abs. [4] Slowly lower your legs down towards the ground, keeping them as straight as possible. Before they touch the ground, stop and hold for a second. [5] Pulling through your toes, slowly bring your legs back up so they are pointing straight up in the air.

Lateral jumps
30sec ON / 15sec REST

[1] Start with your feet hip-width apart and your arms by your sides. [2] Lower yourself down into a half-squat, reaching forward with your arms as you do. [3] Drive up, swing your arms back past your hips and leap as far to your left as you can. [4] Land with soft knees, dropping straight back down into a half-squat. [5] This time when you drive back up, leap as far to your right as you can.

> **Repeat this exercise but for 30sec on and 30sec rest.**

Prone upper-body snow angels
30sec ON / 15sec REST

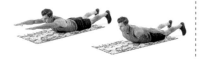

[1] Lie on your stomach with your arms stretched out above your head. [2] Lift your arms and chest off the ground, keeping your toes in contact with the ground. [3] Keeping your arms off the ground, swing them wide around your body until your hands touch your hips. [4] Keep your arms and chest up as you swing your arms back above your head.

Flutter kicks
50sec ON / 10sec REST

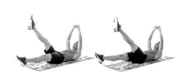

[1] Lie on your back and bring your knees up to your chest. [2] Reach your arms up towards the ceiling, squeezing your rib cage towards your pelvis and curling your shoulder blades off the ground. [3] Keeping your stomach tight, extend your legs and start kicking as if you were doing backstroke. Keep your knees straight. When you reach the end of the set, bend your knees before you lower your feet to the ground.

High heel taps
30sec ON / 15sec REST

[1] Stand in front of a step or something similar that is about 20 cm (8 inches) high. [2] Rest the back of your right heel on the edge of the step, with your weight on your left leg. [3] Jump up and switch legs so that you are now standing on your right leg and the back of your left heel is resting on the step.

> **Repeat this exercise but for 30sec on and 30sec rest.**

STRONGER, FITTER, FASTER, LEANER – HOW GOOD DOES IT FEEL?

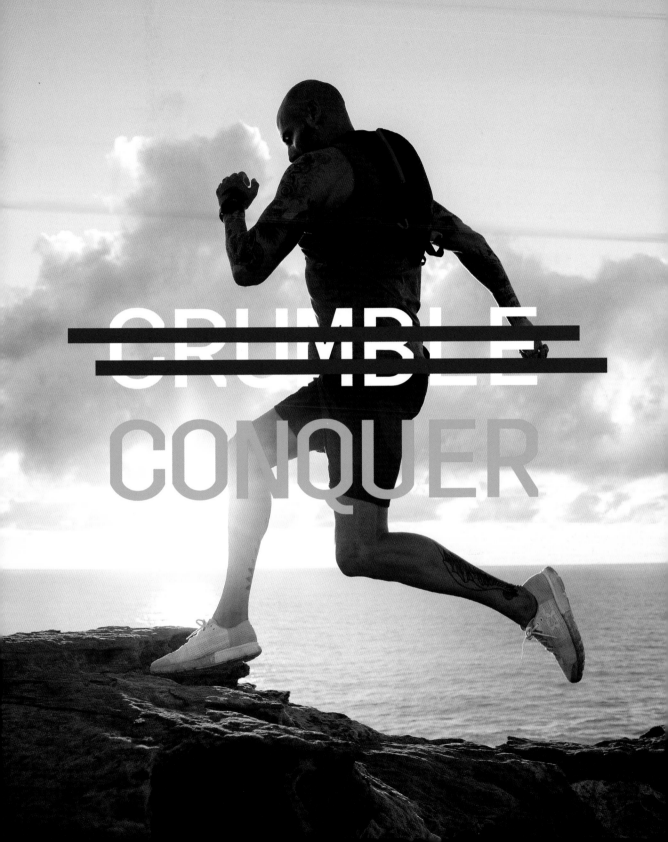

~~CRUMBLE~~

CONQUER

THE
WEEKS//

WEEK 8

WEEK 7

WEEK 6

WEEK 5

WEEK 4

WEEK 3

WEEK 2

WEEK 1 *LET'S GET STARTED!*

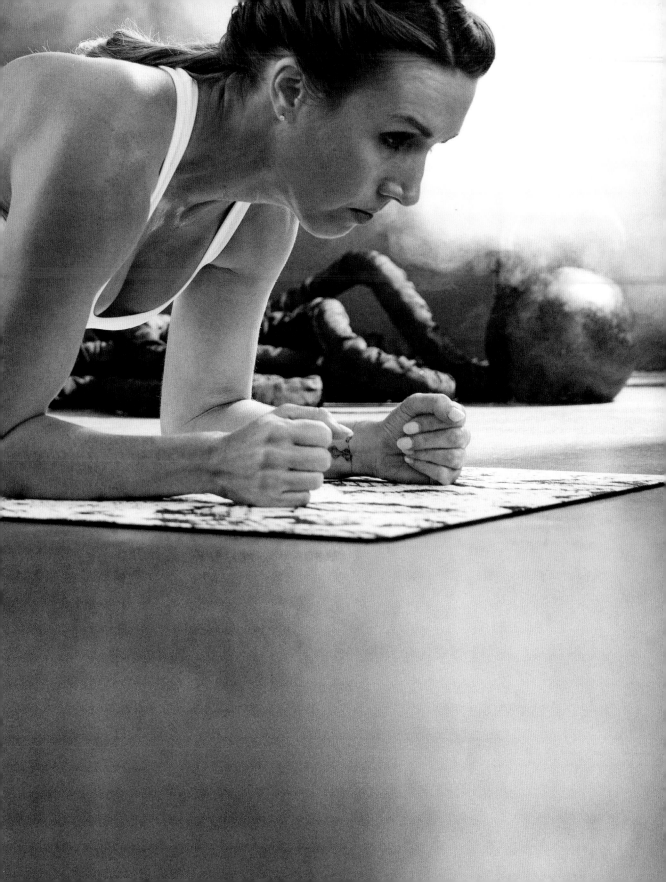

TRANSFORMATION STORIES
CHRISTINA'S STORY

Name: Christina Ratnasinghe

Age: 26

Occupation: Lawyer

When did you complete the 8WTW program? March 2017

What motivated you to undertake this program?
After years of trying to lose weight on my own and without any success, I decided it was time to seek help from the fitness professionals. Having read numerous 8WTW transformation stories online, I knew this was the right program for me.

What goals did you set for yourself?
At first it was about weight loss. I was very self-conscious and had low self-esteem. Halfway through the 8WTW program, it became more about feeling happy with myself and adapting to a healthy lifestyle in the long term.

Did you meet those goals?
Yes! I met and exceeded my personal goals from the 8WTW program.

Which aspect of the program did you find the most challenging?
The workouts for sure! It only became more challenging as the weeks went by. I was always pushing myself harder than the previous day.

Which week was the hardest for you? Why?
Week 2. I found myself craving foods that weren't on the list at the time. I had to stay strong and focus on my goals and remind myself why I started the 8WTW program.

Favourite exercise from the workouts?
I absolutely loved working out with weights – especially the Arnold press with dumbbells. I always looked forward to working on my shoulders.

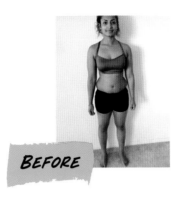

BEFORE

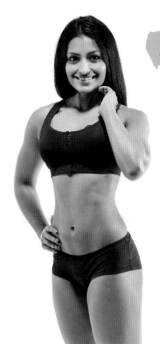

AFTER

Which exercise did you dread the most?

Two-handed dumbbell bent over row. As much as I acknowledge how important working on my back was, this was the exercise I dreaded the most.

Did you discover any new favourite foods?

Absolutely – protein pizza! I'm still enjoying it on the weekends. You just need to be creative with your toppings.

How did you stay motivated on hard days?

With the support of my partner. He always believed in me and my potential. He enjoyed the 8WTW meals as much as I did!

What is your top tip for someone just starting?

Believe in yourself, stay positive and spend time around those who understand and will support you through your life-changing journey.

CHIEF AND EM ARE THE MOST INSPIRING PEOPLE I HAVE MET IN MY LIFE. THEY TRULY LEAD BY EXAMPLE.

WELCOME TO WEEK 1

So, here you are. You've made a decision to make a change, health-wise. Well done! We're about to embark upon a journey to change not only your physical health, but your mindset, diet and complete outlook on health and fitness. It may feel like you are taking a huge step today, but the biggest and most amazing changes happen by putting one foot in front of the other and taking one step at a time.

If you feel a little nervous, just remember that so many people have undertaken this process before you, all with different goals and aspirations. Your goal, just like you, is unique. Where do you see yourself at the end of this program? What's your ultimate body goal? Got it fixed firmly in your head? Good. Write it down, then put it somewhere you'll see and read it every day. Stick it to your bathroom mirror or under your computer screen, or pop it in your wallet or handbag. Just make sure it's easily accessible for those times when you are questioning why you started, or are lacking motivation. You're bound to have those moments, but reminding yourself why you want this, and how you want to look and feel at the end can be very powerful ways to get yourself back on track.

The key to success is to constantly remind yourself of the end goal. You might be a long-term goal person or a step-by-stepper – there are so many

different ways to succeed. We just need to find *your* way, so that in 8 weeks' time, you're exactly where you want to be: a stronger, fitter, healthier and happier version of you.

EMBRACE YOUR NEW DIET

I try to live by the motto, 'you are what you eat'. And I would rather be clean, lean and fresh, than fast, greasy and fatty! Don't get me wrong, we all have our vices and love foods that may not be the best for us (pizza, anyone? Burger?). Food is a touchpoint. It brings back childhood memories and complex issues from our teenage years, or simply makes our tastebuds sing. And that's absolutely fine. We aren't going to remove your favourite foods from your life entirely. We're just going to get you to look at them a little differently. In 8 weeks' time you might find you have a new favourite food or 'vice'. Generally, when we think about dieting (even the word makes me shudder), the vision that pops into our minds is not a good one. But with our program, there are so many recipe options that you shouldn't feel too restricted or like you aren't eating delicious food. Some people even tell us that there are too many food options to choose from. I bet you never thought that would be possible on a diet, did you?

READY? THEN LET'S GET STARTED.

TAKE YOUR MEASUREMENTS

This might not be a fun step, but it's an important one. Tracking your numbers on this journey is going to be vital to your motivation, your dedication and your enthusiasm. Taking measurements is the most honest and true record of your progress, and there's nothing like seeing those numbers change to keep you pushing through the weeks.

These are the important figures to take note of:
[A] Dress/pants size:
[B] Chest:
[C] Waist:
[D] Hips:
[E] Thighs:

Write down your measurements before you start day one of this program, because you're going to start noticing changes quickly. We also want you to take a few 'before' photos. Get down to your underwear (or go *au naturel*, if that's your thing) and ask your partner/mum/mate to take the photos, or set the timer function on your phone's

camera. You want three photos: one from the front, one from the side and one from the back. It might not be fun to look at those right now, but keep visualising where you'll be after 8 weeks. Print these out, then put them into an envelope in a safe place. Trust me, you'll be glad you have them 8 weeks from now.

You might be wondering why we haven't asked you to weigh yourself. It's because your weight doesn't matter for this program. These measurements and your photos will be enough. Trust us!

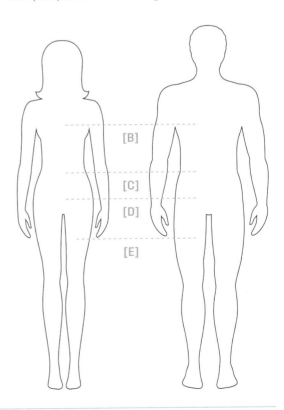

STOP AND THINK

It's a good idea to think of this eating plan as a reboot rather than a diet. Making changes is definitely hard, but try to focus on what you will have at the end of the 8 weeks as your biggest reward. You're teaching your body how to use food for the right reasons again. Your body probably knew how to do it once, but it forgot along the way, when all the healthier choices that your parents made for you became your responsibility. That's why diets don't work – they have a start and a finish. This plan, however, is a foundation for what comes next.

How often do you open the fridge when you aren't hungry, search through it and then eat something simply because you're bored? We've all done it, but we're going to work on eliminating that habit. We want you to try to do something else – make a cup of tea or coffee, make a phone call or step outside for some fresh air. Try not to let a habitual food temptation trip you up every time.

So take a moment to stop and think: how can you start to choose healthier options that you will look forward to eating? Eat slowly and enjoy the taste. A salad will still taste good after an hour on your plate. Fast food tastes stale and almost old once it gets cold or sits on your plate for that same hour.

WHAT TO EXPECT

Week 1 will be a shock. Even if you already have a good, balanced diet and enjoy a rigorous exercise routine, it's going to challenge you because it's different from what you usually do. The hardest part of any new routine is the first 2 weeks. Drinking more water, changing your eating habits, exercising and forgoing everyday treats can be tough. But if you can do it for 5 to 10 days straight, you can make a real difference straight out of the starting gates.

The challenges you face when it comes to food will depend on your personality type; you might have to curb your sweet tooth or avoid the salty snacks you love. You might be an emotional eater, or stress might make you lose your appetite. When you face temptation, remind yourself why you're doing this, and that this program is not just about the food. It's about creating healthy new habits, finding new hobbies and fitness activities to enjoy, and discovering new healthier meals.

Every person reacts differently to our program. You might find that it makes you feel slow or lethargic, or maybe a little bit weak. Or, you may notice an increase in energy. However you feel is fine. Listen to your body and give it the extra support it needs to get through this challenging time – that might be drinking more water, getting to bed earlier or having a healthy snack. Just try to stick to the program as much as you can. Your body and mind are smart – they're used to a routine, and you are probably dramatically changing the routine they have been used to for many years. Building new habits will take time. If you have to ask yourself one question each day, let it be this: 'Is it on The List?' (see the next page). If it isn't, don't eat it!

FOLLOW THESE RULES IN WEEK 1 AND BEYOND

+ You must drink 2 litres (70 fl oz/8 cups) of water each day, without fail. Either have 2 glasses of water with each meal, or sip 2–3 litres (70–105 fl oz/8–12 cups) throughout the day. Try not to go over 4 litres (140 fl oz/ 16 cups) unless you already drink this much. It's definitely possible to drink too much water, and that carries its own set of risks. We're aiming for maximum hydration without putting your system at risk.

+ You must eat your 'Compulsory daily greens' (see The List on page 76). Compulsory means you need it and you have to have it! Roughage ensures your metabolism and body are working at their best. The 100–150 g (3½–5½ oz) for women and 150–200 g (5½–7 oz) for men of salad roughage every day is compulsory. You'll learn to love it for the way it makes you feel. It might seem like a lot of leaves to begin with, but the salads you can make for lunch and dinner are ridiculously good – just use your imagination. Salads and greens are delicious when prepared well.

+ As a general rule of thumb, you don't want to eat more than 30–50 g (1–1 ¾ oz) of carbs in a single day for the entire first week. This is simply a guideline, for the time being. Carbs are not the enemy – they serve many beneficial purposes. However, if you're like the majority of people who eat a 'Western' diet, it is very likely that you've been consuming them in far greater quantities than necessary. This first week is all about reminding your body how to use carbs – the right way. By greatly reducing them in their complex form (but not eliminating them entirely) in the first week, your body will start fuelling itself in a much more efficient manner. Stick with it – you can do it!

+ Ladies, unless you are very tall and have a large frame, you should never be eating as much as your boyfriend, husband or other men. Women are smaller and they simply don't need the same amount of food.

+ Try to exercise 6 days out of every 7. It doesn't matter which day you have off – do whatever works best for your schedule. For example, work out every day from Monday to Saturday, then have a rest on Sunday. But you must have a complete day off from exercise once a week. A walk or a gentle swim on your rest day is fine, but try not to wear yourself out. Your body can only get stronger when it has the chance to recover, and it needs time to repair.

THE LIST: *WEEK 1*

For the next 8 weeks, these pages will be your food compass. Never eat until you're full, just until you're satisfied. As of this week, you can eat everything on the next couple of pages.

COMPULSORY GREENS ('SALAD ROUGHAGE')

 150 g (5½ oz) every day

 200 g (7 oz) every day

You need to eat the amounts we've specified to ensure you're getting enough fibre and visiting the restroom for the right reasons. If you eat this quantity, you won't need any extra fibre supplements.

In Weeks 1 and 2, only eat these 5 greens.

+ Baby English spinach
+ Celery (you can have an unlimited amount every day)
+ Cucumber (you can have an unlimited amount every day)
+ Lettuce (all types)
+ Watercress

VEGETABLES

 150 g (5½ oz) every day

 200 g (7 oz) every day

For Weeks 1 and 2, eat ONLY the vegies listed here in addition to the compulsory greens (see left).

+ Asparagus
+ Avocado (no more than ¼ avocado per day)
+ Bean sprouts
+ Bok choy (pak choy)
+ Capsicum (pepper)
+ Chinese cabbage (wong bok)
+ Eggplant (aubergine)
+ English spinach (fresh or frozen)
+ Fennel
+ Mushrooms
+ Okra
+ Onion
+ Radish
+ Spring onion (scallion)
+ Tomato (no more than ½ medium tomato or 6 cherry tomatoes per day)
+ Zucchini (courgette)

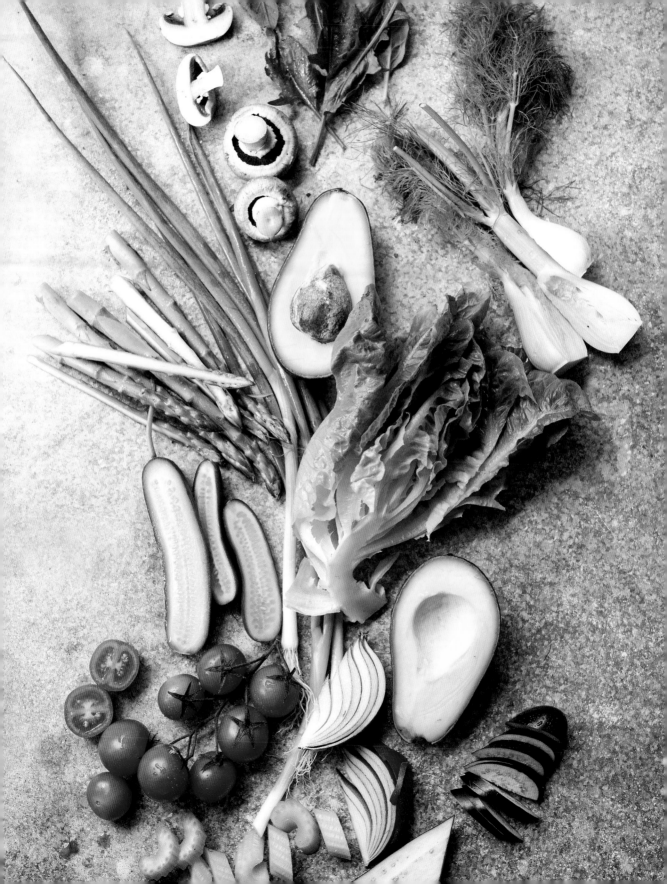

MEATS AND SEAFOOD

Men and women: a portion about the size of your palm per meal – anything from 200–300 g (7–10½ oz) . You can have 3 serves a day.

+ Beef: lean cuts, veal or minced* (ground)
+ Chicken: lean meat or minced* (ground) only – no skin, no wings, no stuffing, not fried, no sauce (Nando's or Oporto chicken with no sauce is fine)
+ Fish: any fresh, frozen or tinned (if tinned, in springwater or brine only)
+ Kangaroo and kangaroo sausages
+ Lamb: very lean cuts
+ Pork: very lean cuts, including low-fat ham, trimmed bacon and shoulder bacon
+ Seafood: any fresh, frozen or tinned (in springwater or brine only), including shellfish and crustaceans
+ Smoked salmon
+ Turkey: lean meat or minced* (ground) only – no skin or wings

*Minced (ground) meats must be under 8% fat.

HEAD TO THE RECIPES FOR WEEK 1 ON PAGE 134.

DAIRY AND EGGS

+ Cheeses: only fat-free or very low fat cheese products, such as cottage cheese, cream cheese (5% fat), extra light ricotta cheese, quark, light shredded cheese (no more than a snack-tub size, i.e. less than 30 g/1 oz per day)
+ Egg whites (unlimited)
+ Egg yolks (no more than 2 per day)
+ Milk: skim or fat-free/non-fat (up to 300 ml/ 10½ fl oz per day)
+ Non-dairy milks: unsweetened low-fat or skim soy milk or unsweetened almond milk
+ Sour cream: only fat-free or very low-fat (no more than 30 g/1 oz per day)
+ Yoghurt: 1 serve per day of low-fat, low-carb, low-sugar plain or vanilla yoghurt (under 6 g sugar per serve)

BREADS, NOODLES AND GRAINS

You can have 1 serve per day

+ Two 3 mm (⅛ inch) thick slices of Protein bread from The Protein Bread Co. (theproteinbreadco.com.au) – best toasted
+ 1 pizza base from The Protein Bread Co. (go easy on the cheese)
+ Konjac, shirataki or Slendier noodles (found in the health food aisle of the supermarket and Asian grocery stores)
+ Konjac rice

HERBS, SPICES AND KEY INGREDIENTS

+ Black pepper (freshly ground)
+ Canola oil spray (use sparingly, and not in all recipes)
+ Chia seeds
+ Chilli: fresh red/green chilli, chilli flakes, ancho chilli, smoked chipotle chilli
+ Chlorophyll (best in liquid form and very important for a healthy gut)
+ Curry paste and powder
+ Dried spices (essentials are paprika, roast vegetable seasoning and Asian spice blends)
+ French shallots
+ Garlic
+ Ginger
+ Herbs (fresh and dried)
+ Lemon juice
+ Lemongrass
+ Lime juice
+ Linseed (flaxseed) oil
+ Mustard
+ Nori sheets
+ Protein powder
+ Salt-reduced soy sauce
+ Sea salt
+ Stock: low-sodium liquid stock and stock (bouillon) cubes
+ Sugar-free chewing gum
+ Sugar-free non-fat cocoa powder
+ Sugar-free sweeteners: e.g. stevia, Splenda, Equal (use as little as possible)
+ Tabasco sauce
+ Vanilla extract
+ Vinegar: apple cider, balsamic, white
+ Vitamin B supplement or Berocca

DRINKS

+ Water (up to 3 litres/105 fl oz per day)
+ Coffee (up to 3 per day if made with water, only 1 per day if made with steamed skim or fat-free milk and no water; you can add sweeteners from The List)
+ Tea and herbal tea (up to 3 per day; you can add sweeteners from The List, as well as skim or fat-free milk)
+ Fresh ginger tea – fantastic for easing stomach upsets or headaches
+ Sugar-free hot chocolate (no more than 1 per day)

A GOOD FRYING PAN WILL MAKE A WORLD OF DIFFERENCE, AND A GEORGE FOREMAN GRILL IS EVEN BETTER. YOU NEED TO DRY-FRY YOUR FOOD IN ITS OWN JUICES RATHER THAN ADDING OIL OR BUTTER.

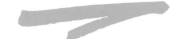

WEEK 8

WEEK 7

WEEK 6

WEEK 5

WEEK 4

WEEK 3

WEEK 2

YOU'RE ON YOUR WAY!

WEEK 1

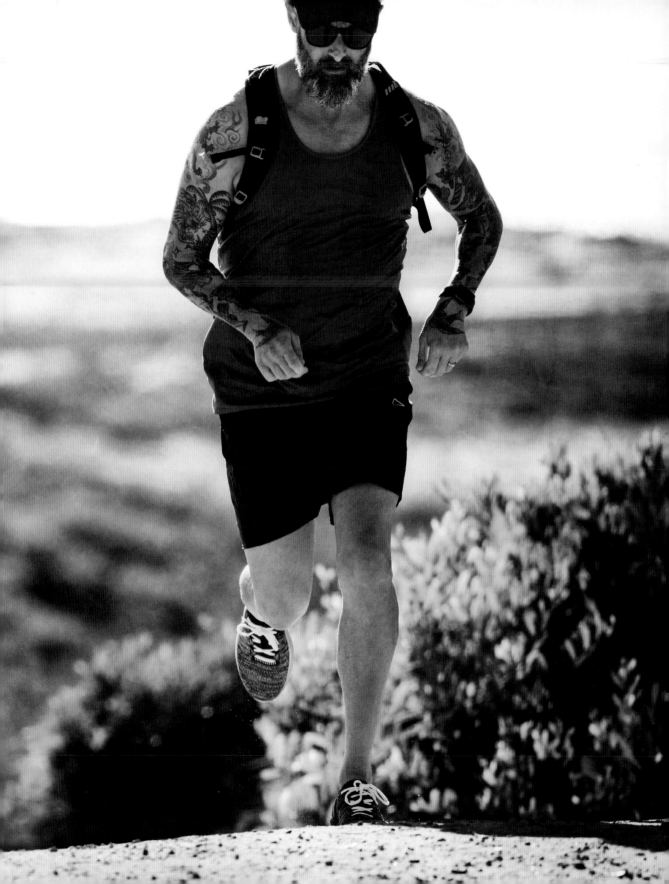

TRANSFORMATION STORIES
ANDY'S STORY

Name: Andy Anastasi

Age: 43

Occupation: Technology Manager

When did you complete the 8WTW program? December 2017

What motivated you to undertake this program?
I was sitting in a doctor's surgery about to have a colonoscopy for suspect growths in my colon. I was flicking through a magazine and saw Guy Sebastian's transformation. I thought, 'There's no way this is fake or photoshopped.' I needed to make some lifestyle changes across my health and fitness. I'd had enough of fad diets and workouts.

What goals did you set for yourself?
My first goal was to commit to the 2 weeks of no sugar/no alcohol, and as the weeks progressed, my other goals were focused around ensuring I prepped my meals for 5 days of the week and ran 1 mile in under 7 minutes (my first attempt was about 14 minutes). Lastly, I wanted to be comfortable with my appearance in the mirror.

Did you meet those goals?
Smashed them!

Which aspect of the program did you find the most challenging?
The first 2 weeks were the most challenging, as portion control and diet were changed – with removing breads, pastas and sugars . Walking down the middle aisle of any supermarket was a struggle, so I opted to carry a cucumber or celery stick with me and whenever the urge struck, I ate that.

Which week was the hardest for you? Why?
Week 2 because I had just completed a week of the new diet and was struggling mentally on how I would smash it for another 7 weeks. Thankfully, the reinforcement messages from Em on a regular basis helped motivate me to continue and stay focused, creating a good discipline that I've taken beyond the 8 weeks.

Favourite exercise from the workouts?
Anything with a dumbbell and a shoulder exercise.

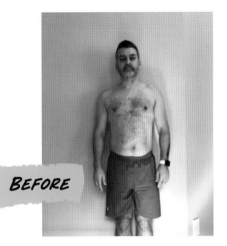

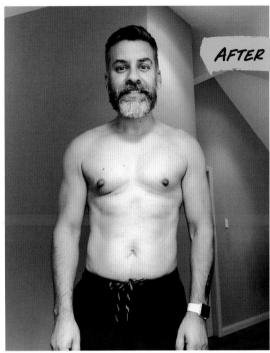

I absolutely loved the core workouts as, unlike other times I'd done core sessions, these workouts were designed in a way that focused on the muscle group and when I worked on my core I felt it the next day. I call that 'the good pain'.

Which exercise did you dread the most?

The first couple of weeks I dreaded any squat, especially a pike squat. We've now come to respect one another.

Did you discover any new favourite foods?

Plenty – from loving the various ways I could make a salad feel meaty enough to be a main meal, to Protein Bread Company bread that didn't give me the standard carb bloat, and konjac noodles, spaghetti and lasagne.

How did you stay motivated on hard days?

What initially motivated me was the article on Guy's transformation. So at first, it was about going back to that article. From there, I looked at what I called my 'fat' photos and reminded myself that this would be the last time I'd look like that. Sharing my food pics with other individuals on their journey was a great opportunity to talk to people I knew were going through the same journey and struggles as I was. It was easy to find new motivation as Em would also send weekly messages of encouragement and motivation to keep us focused. As time went by, it was more about remaining disciplined.

What is your top tip for someone just starting?

This is for people who are ready to commit to a real lifestyle change and who've had enough of sitting on the couch thinking, 'I can't do this.' If you are looking for an opportunity to change your life in a way that gives you the tools, support mechanism and education around improving your fitness and nutrition after 8 short weeks, this is it.

WELCOME TO WEEK 2

Welcome to your second week! Think about these weeks as if you are filling up a water balloon. Each day that you stick to the plan, you are filling the balloon a little more. If you break the rules, it's like bursting that water balloon and having to start all over again. Believe in yourself and you can survive this!

I hope you got through the week unscathed, and feel stronger for doing so. The program is helping you take just a few steps at a time to a different way of thinking, eating and generally being. A good way to reassess is to remember why you started 8WTW. What made you pick up this book? Think about the progress you have made in just one week and how much of a difference a solid week of determination can make.

DEALING WITH SLIP-UPS

Don't worry if you had any little slip-ups like missing a workout or eating something that wasn't on The List. We aren't here to punish you for being human. If it happens often, you probably need to take a look at why it's happening – is it peer pressure? Are you emotionally wrung-out or fed up? Was it an accident (this happens), or are there other reasons? If there are deeper reasons for your behaviour, the sooner you can identify those and address any feelings connected to them, the faster you'll be able to learn to control them. And once you can control your emotions and how they cause you to act, you will make progress. Give yourself time to think all this through, then tell yourself that you CAN do this! I find I'm more inclined to do something when I write it down or say it out loud as a mantra – perhaps that will work for you too.

TIP: WE OFTEN DON'T REALISE WE'RE DEHYDRATED UNTIL WE'RE REALLY DEHYDRATED. STAYING HYDRATED CAN MEAN YOU HAVE THE EXTRA PUSH THAT'S GOING TO GET YOU TO THAT LAST REP OR SPRINT IN CHIEF'S WORKOUTS. SO DRINK UP!

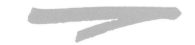

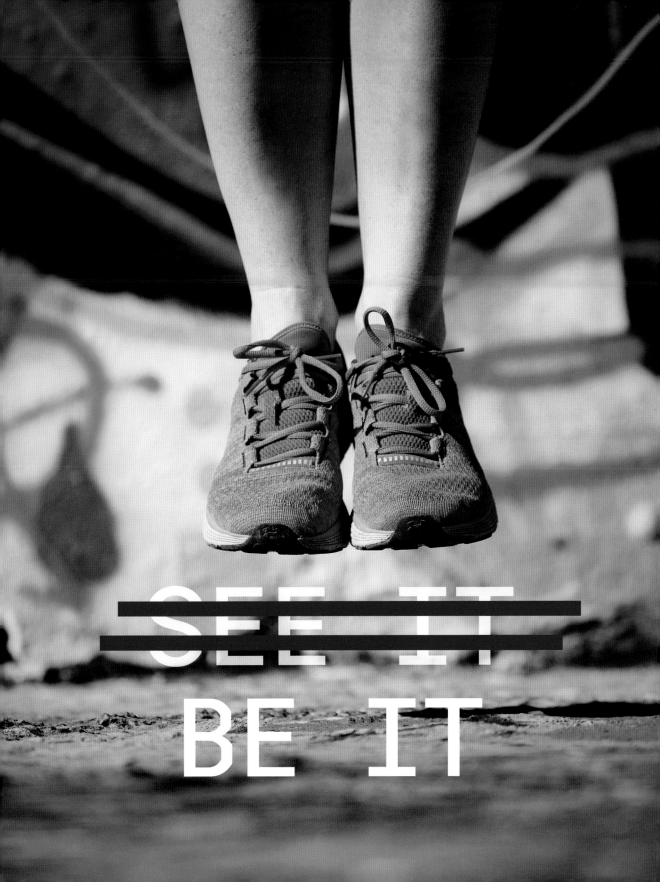

SEE IT

BE IT

SLEEP

I love sleep. I don't get enough of it (who does?), but I do try my best to ensure that the shut-eye I get is quality rest time.

It's a little-known fact that one of the most important keys to fat loss and living a healthy life is getting the right amount of sleep. We often hear about drinking enough water, getting enough exercise and eating the right foods (and that's just from me!), but sleep is the true 'elixir' of vitality. It's the glue that holds it all together.

Don't get me wrong: everyone has a restless night every now and then, and that's completely normal. But when bad sleep turns into a habit, it can wreak havoc on your ability to function on a day-to-day basis.

I have read so many research papers about the effects of not getting enough sleep and they all draw the same conclusion: you could be putting yourself at risk for impaired glucose tolerance (leading to Type 2 diabetes), hypertension, high blood pressure, depression and weight gain. Lack of sleep can play a huge part in hindering your weight loss and fat loss. Without adequate sleep, your moods can change, you won't be able to do your job properly and you definitely won't be the first person on the list when your friends are looking for a fun night out.

It's important to get rid of any bad habits that have crept in and are affecting your quality and quantity of sleep, and replace them with good habits. Good habits will have you waking up a minute before your alarm clock sounds, raring and ready to go, and not wanting to crawl under your desk for a nap at 3pm.

We all suffer from stress in one way or another, and it can have a big impact on your sleep. You may notice it more in the form of weird dreams at the beginning of this transformation. You may continue to have those unexplainable dreams – they are just your mind working through the day's events, thoughts, stresses and so on.

HERE ARE A FEW SIMPLE WAYS TO NURTURE GOOD SLEEP HABITS

+ Get yourself into the right routine. This one is going to be the hardest for parents, but you need to really set yourself a rule. If you don't usually go to bed until later in the evening, try to start going to bed 20–30 minutes earlier every week. The aim is to find a bedtime that leads to feeling refreshed and revitalised when you wake up. Once you find that bedtime, stick to it (or as close to it as possible). That way your body and mind will know that it is time to wind down and prepare for some quality rest.

+ Try not to eat for at least an hour before you go to bed. When you lie down, the acids in your stomach level out, which means that heartburn and indigestion may come on. You want to avoid anything that makes it hard to switch off. Eating also increases your metabolism, which can sometimes raise your heart rate and energy levels. Also, try not to have that nightcap of alcohol. It may help you get off to sleep, but after those initial effects wear off, it can prevent you from getting the deep, restorative sleep you need, so it's not a great habit to keep.

+ Avoid all stimulants after 4pm. Some people swear by herbal teas such as chamomile or peppermint as a relaxing way to wind down before bed.

+ Turn off your phone, or put it on silent. And no social media at bedtime. Give those apps a rest – they'll still be there in the morning.

If you've followed all of these steps and you still can't sleep, then get up. Don't lie there willing it to happen, because it probably won't and you'll just be adding to your stress bucket. Get up and read a book for 20 minutes, then try again.

A NOTE ON THE WORKOUTS FOR THIS WEEK

As well as the long-term goals I set for myself, I like to set myself up with some weekly goals.

These could be as simple as making sure I do push-ups every day and logging my workout times so I can reassess them later when I'm feeling superhuman (in about 8 weeks' time). Do whatever works for you to help you feel both energised and motivated to stay on track.

Look at Chief's DARC workouts again now (see page 34), and get cracking on a fantastic start to Week 2.

THE LIST: WEEK 2

This week you will continue to follow The List from Week 1 (pages 76–79). We will add new foods every 2 weeks until we're back to healthier options and carbs, but you'll see that there are a few exceptions as you work through the book. We want to make your body and mind function a lot better and more clearly, and this is part of the process.

I hope that you are loving the recipes (there are new recipes for this week on page 144), and that you are coming up with your own amazing dishes using the ingredients on The List. You may even have created your new favourite lunch, dinner or snack. You can look forward to adding more ingredients to the mix in Week 3.

GOOD LUCK!

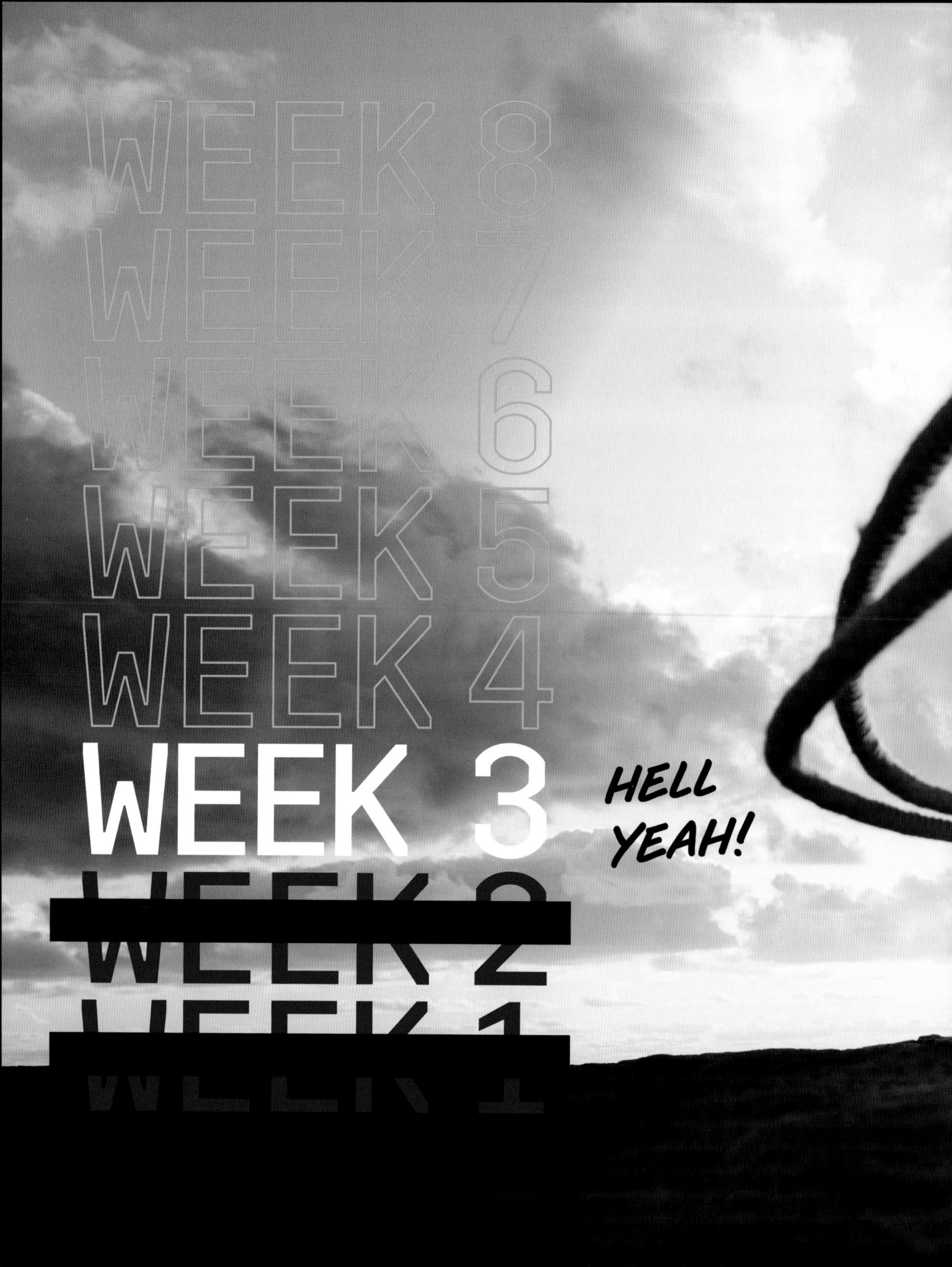
WEEK 8
WEEK 7
WEEK 6
WEEK 5
WEEK 4
WEEK 3
HELL YEAH!
~~WEEK 2~~
~~WEEK 1~~

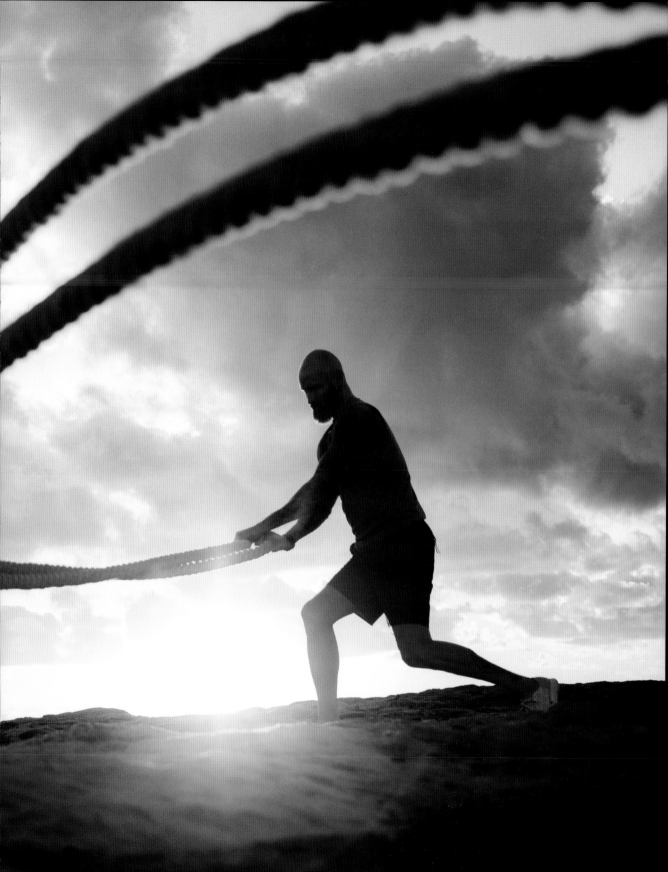

TRANSFORMATION STORIES
RICHARD & REBECCA'S STORY

Name: Richard & Rebecca Wokes

Age: 39 & 41

Occupations: Richard is Head of Operations at Sony PlayStation
Rebecca is NSW Retail State Manager at Colonial First State

When did you complete the 8WTW program? First time was
October 2013 (we've done it a few times!)

What motivated you to undertake this program?
Richard: My wife and I had been training for a while. Although we were fit, we wanted to up our performance.

Rebecca: The first time I did the program it was to help me get back into a fitness regime after baby number two. I was struggling, and finding time and motivation was challenging. I couldn't shift the baby weight. And I signed up to do the program again after that first round because I saw the improvements on my performance and fitness.

What goals did you set for yourself?
Richard: There weren't necessarily any weight loss or muscle gain goals. At our stage of our training it was more about feeling faster, fitter, stronger. Shredding was just a by-product of the discipline the program provided.

Rebecca: I agree. Though first time around, my goal was about dropping weight and toning up.

Did you meet those goals?
Rebecca: Yes. The first time around, I was high-fiving myself at the 2-week point. The results were incredible! I just felt amazing.

Which aspect of the program did you find the most challenging?
Richard: Finding time to prepare the meals and give us some variety was challenging. So was getting used to the portion sizes.

Which week was the hardest for you? Why?
Richard: The first couple of weeks are always the hardest as your body is getting used to the eating plan and with three young kids, a glass of wine is always close at hand, so you miss that. But once the first couple of weeks are done, it just becomes the norm. Four years later, the lessons we learned on the plan are still very much a part of our diet. Well, maybe a glass of wine has been re-introduced.

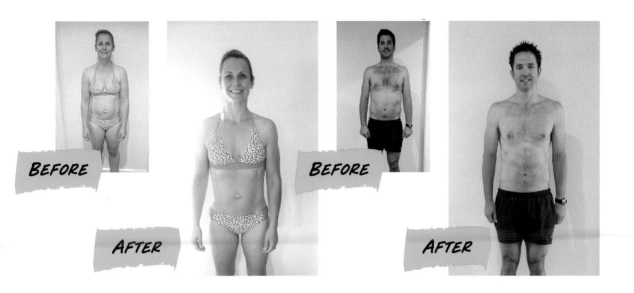

BEFORE

AFTER

BEFORE

AFTER

Favourite exercise from the workouts?
Richard: I don't think there is one favourite exercise or one I dread the most. We go to Em and Chief's Original Bootcamp to get pushed, and the motto 'no pain, no gain' is something, as a family, we understand.

Did you discover any new favourite foods?
Rebecca: Zoodles (zucchini noodles) have become a great alternative to pasta, and the kids love them! And breakfast muffins are great to make and eat on the run, which is pretty much the case for us most mornings.

How did you stay motivated on hard days?
Richard: When you start seeing results after 2 weeks, it makes it easier to keep motivated. That, and the crew at Original Bootcamp who continually push you to get the best out of yourselves make it possible – not easy, but possible. Doing the program

with my wife meant that we were both going through it together. That made a huge difference as we were able to remove the temptations together.

What is your top tip for someone just starting?
Rebecca: Stick with it, surround yourself with like-minded people for the 8 weeks and you will see the results. And not just in your waist, but your whole fitness levels will reach a new height.

STICK WITH IT, SURROUND YOURSELF WITH LIKE-MINDED PEOPLE FOR THE 8 WEEKS AND YOU WILL SEE THE RESULTS.

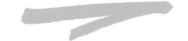

WELCOME TO WEEK 3

We're entering Week 3 already – wow! I hope you're starting to feel
fantastic and can already see the changes. Are you focusing on your goals?

THE RECIPES

All the recipes in this book are suitable for the
entire 8WTW program, working backwards. This
means that you can use any of the recipes from
the previous weeks. Given that you're in Week 3,
you can also choose from the recipes from Week 1
and Week 2. I have no doubt that you've also come
up with some amazing recipes yourself. I know this
because so many of our 8WTW participants have
created their own favourite meals from The List.
At 8WTW HQ, we have an archive of over 1500
recipes, which is growing every day.

The meals and snacks that you have on this
program can be as fancy or as simple as you like.
It really depends on how adventurous you are
in the kitchen, whether you have the extra time
to spend there and how much you know about
flavours and food. Me? I know my way around the
kitchen, but Hubby is my masterchef!

This week, we're going to add some new ingredients
to keep your food interesting and make sure we're
building up your metabolism and new body in the
right way. I bet you never thought you'd be excited
about vegetables! Remember, food is not the
enemy. Just make sure that whatever you eat is
earned, used or eaten in the right way, as well as
in the right amounts. Don't forget to watch your
portion sizes – eat small amounts, and eat slowly.

If you haven't found anything you really enjoy yet,
look over The List again, or look through all the
recipes for inspiration. You don't want to think
of these foods as 'diet' foods. You want to find
a way to enjoy them long after this 8-week
program is complete. Finding foods that you can
enjoy as healthier options is the perfect habit to
form over the next few weeks, so that choosing
healthier options becomes second nature to you.

GOALS

Statistics prove that it is easier to stick with something if you have more than one goal. Think about the goals you set at the beginning of the program. Can you break them down into smaller goals? We all have a picture in our heads of the best version of ourselves. If your goal is about your size, try not to imagine a goal weight so much as a goal size. A measuring tape is going to be a more powerful indicator of your success than the scales. The other side of that goal might focus on something active – something you want to be good at. If you aren't really into fitness, don't care for running or lifting a certain weight, focus instead on one thing that you would like to change in your everyday life. It could be something as simple as making sure that you walk a certain distance each day or preparing your work lunch the day before. Little steps at a time will help you reach whatever your larger goal might be.

SCALES VERSUS MEASURING TAPE

If you're used to weighing yourself, you may be grumbling that you *have* to weigh yourself, and that it's just how you are. But I'm pretty sure that most people would be upset by the number on the scales at least once a week. You might feel disappointment because you aren't a certain number, anger because you worked so hard (and that can't be defined by a number) and maybe a little disillusioned that your body isn't doing what you want it to do. First and foremost: you should never let the scales dictate your worth.

You are more than that number flashing back at you. Don't beat yourself up about a number that means so little.

When I stick to the 8WTW eating plan, I drop a dress size or more. How do I know? My tape measure tells me so. Do I ever drop any weight? I don't know, and I don't care.

THE DAY I STOPPED WEIGHING MYSELF, ABOUT 15 YEARS AGO, WAS THE BEST DAY. I STOPPED STRESSING ABOUT 'LOSING WEIGHT', AND STARTED WORKING ON GETTING FIT AND BEING HEALTHY.

I never have to deal with the disappointment of the number on the scales not being what magazines and Google tell me it should be, and I feel a lot better for it.

So, ditch your scales and stick with the measuring tape. You'll be able to accurately track your progress in terms of size simply by measuring the same places on your body and keeping records. Admittedly, this isn't a great tool if you want to figure out your body fat (you'll need to get out the calipers for that), but it's all you need for measuring your progress on a weekly basis.

NOW, LET'S HIT WEEK 3!

THE LIST: *WEEKS 3 & 4*

This week we are adding some more vegetables to The List and increasing the daily quantity you can eat. You can also enjoy a small handful of natural almonds every second day (e.g. on Tuesday, Thursday and Saturday).

VEGETABLES

 250 g (9 oz) per day

 300 g (10½ oz) per day

Add these to the original list.

+ Broccoli
+ Brussels sprouts
+ Cabbage
+ Carrot
+ Cauliflower
+ Leek
+ Pumpkin (winter squash)
+ Runner beans
+ Squash
+ String beans

NUTS

 1 small handful (10–15 nuts) every second day

 1 small handful (20 nuts) every second day

+ Natural almonds

OIL

+ Coconut oil (1 teaspoon per day); best used when cooking in a frying pan – it tastes amazing!

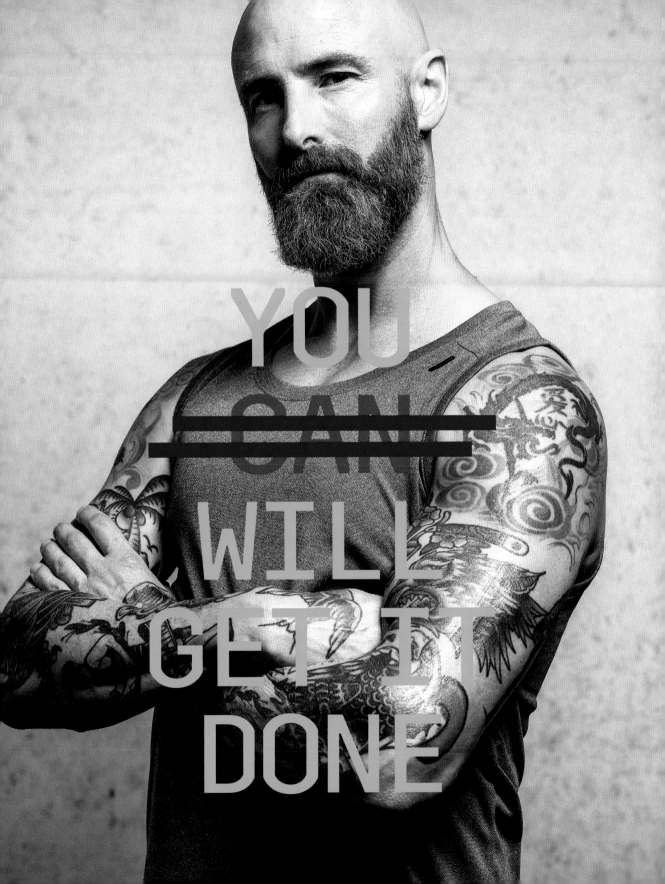

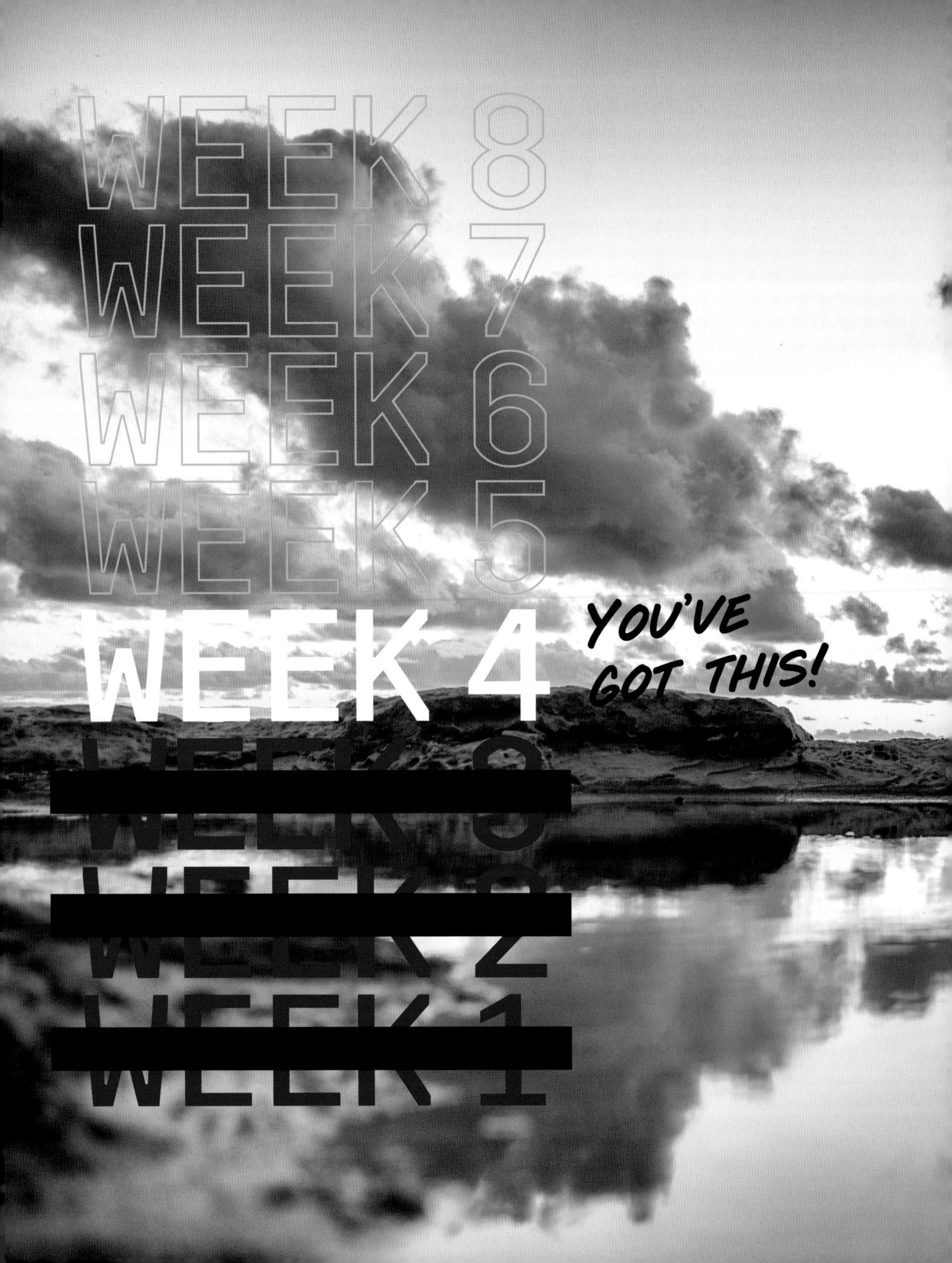
WEEK 8
WEEK 7
WEEK 6
WEEK 5
WEEK 4
YOU'VE GOT THIS!
~~WEEK 3~~
~~WEEK 2~~
~~WEEK 1~~

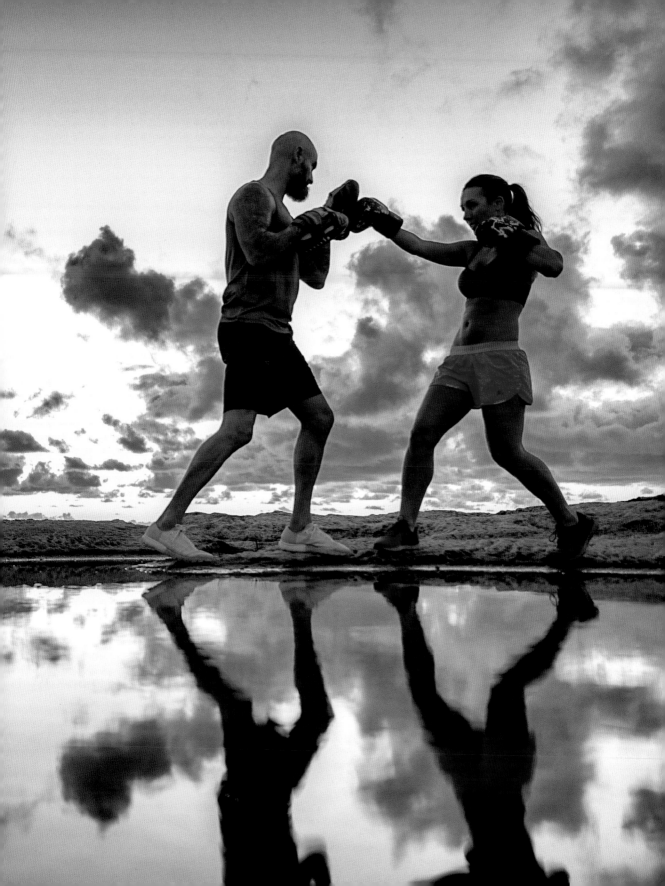

TRANSFORMATION STORIES
SHARLEEN'S STORY

Name: Sharleen Rea

Age: 56

Occupation: IT Program Manager

When did you complete the 8WTW program? 2015 and 2017

What motivated you to undertake this program?
I saw a picture of myself at a family function and realised my weight had crept up way more than I'd thought. My lower back issues were also getting worse. I decided I didn't want to be immobile at such a young age. I knew what it felt like to be fit, and I missed that. I'd started to exercise on my own but wasn't getting anywhere and didn't just want the same old gym-based workouts. A colleague at work suggested Original Bootcamp. He told me about the 8WTW program and the great success people were having with it, but also that it wasn't for the faint-hearted. That turned out to be the best advice ever (thanks, Hany).

What goals did you set for yourself?
I wanted to feel fit and toned – there's a special way your body feels and moves when you are fit. I wanted to be physically stronger. Standing on a set of scales and getting a number was never the goal,

but I wanted to fit in clothes that had been in the back of my closet for years and BUY some new ones! I always work better when there is a specific reason I'm doing something, so I set myself a goal to be able to run a 10 km race and do an obstacle race.

Did you meet those goals?
YES! I ran three 10 km races and did the 9 km Finisher Spartan Race. For me, it was such an achievement because I went from never running to completing four races. Even better, those old clothes in the back of the closet turned out to be too big!

Which aspect of the program did you find the most challenging?
Changing my behaviour. I was a comfort eater. When I got stressed, upset or bored, I'd eat and my go-to food was potato chips, especially Kettle Chips. I could mow through a whole bag without even thinking.

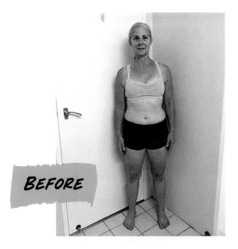

BEFORE

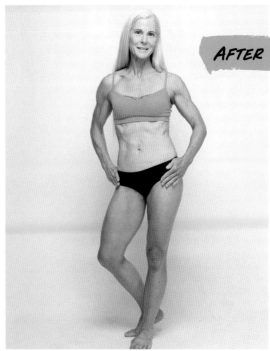

AFTER

Which week was the hardest for you? Why?

I'd say Week 3. The first 2 weeks it's all new and you have motivation, then you hit a wall and you're tired, with no energy and doubt starts to creep in. 'Can I do this for another 5 weeks?' It's the little voice in your head that says, 'Oh, a couple of chips won't matter. A glass of wine is good for me.' All those little justifications ... DON'T LISTEN!

Favourite exercise from the workouts?

Good mornings.

Which exercise did you dread the most?

Push-ups.

Did you discover any new favourite foods?

The Protein Bread Co. products! Making a pizza or nachos with their pizza crust mix is better than anything you could buy. I've even added it to omelettes in the past, and it's delicious!

How did you stay motivated on hard days?

The key is willpower and determination. I was not going to be defeated by a bag of chips or a piece of chocolate. I kept thinking of how much I wanted my goals. Giving up is not in my nature. Em and Chief are always there as inspiration, and Em is good for telling you things straight, like 'Stop being an idiot and just get on with it.'

What is your top tip for someone just starting?

You've got to get your head into it, You have to WANT to achieve your goals. Em and Chief can tell you what to eat and what exercises to do, but it's YOU that has to do the work – no-one else. Make up your mind that you're doing this for yourself, and don't listen to those that start knocking what you are doing. It is a lifestyle change to healthy eating and exercise NOT A DIET! Commit and follow the plan and you will succeed. And one thing to remember is that neither age nor gender matter.

WELCOME TO WEEK 4

Week 4 and still going strong – well done! You're almost halfway through your total body transformation. By this stage, you should have formed new habits that are enjoyable, and noticed a big change in how your clothing fits. Have you also noticed how much better your skin looks, and how much more energy you have?

As humans, we're all different. You might be finding the program easy to stick to, or you might be finding it hard to keep up – because of your old habits, work situations, social occasions or family. Don't beat yourself up about which camp you're in. You're still here, reading this book, which means you're still going, and still chasing your goal.

Remember, there are really only three things you need to master to make the 8WTW program work for you:

[1] Drink 2 litres (70 fl oz/8 cups) of water each day
[2] Exercise 6 days a week
[3] Follow the plan, by sticking to The List of allowed foods

If you give the program a red-hot crack, it's absolutely possible to reach your goal because things get easier as you go along. Willpower is like a muscle: it gets stronger every time you use it.

At this stage of the program, you should start to broaden your diet plan. Eat plenty of different types of vegetables, as well as different proteins, such as chicken and fish. And find some meals that are easy to take to work. If you're cooking for a family, you can serve the same meal to everyone, and simply add some bread or potatoes for the kids or other family members who aren't joining you on this transformation. Do whatever you can to make it easier for you to stick to your goals. It's really that simple.

Remember when you were a kid, and your parents served you chicken and vegetables for dinner? They'd say, 'You aren't leaving the table until it's gone!' You should pretty much be at the same stage now in Week 4 of the plan. Prepare yourself a nice size of your protein of choice, and a good array of colourful vegetables that you enjoy or a big crunchy salad.

WEIGHT LOSS VERSUS FAT LOSS

I've already talked about ditching the scales, but I'm going to harp on about it again. If you're a serial scale hopper, you'll have noticed that the numbers aren't budging nearly as fast as they did in the beginning. That's all right; in fact, it's probably a good thing. Don't worry – you're stripping fat, but building lean muscle, and muscle is heavy.

Your body is a complex machine. On an average day outside of this plan, you feed your body what it needs to keep your eyes open, your brain functioning and your tastebuds happy. Prior to this plan, your food choices were different. The sugar content of your chosen foods would have been much higher (even if you were eating fruit and smoothies), and that's what made your blood sugar spike up and down. Remember the 3pm lull at the office, when you'd tell yourself that you deserved a little treat? Or partook in the office birthday cake or hit the cookie jar? That was your body telling you *more sugar!*, because that's what you were used to. It was a habit.

So, any tiredness that you may or may not be feeling can simply be put down to the fact that you're not used to fuelling your body in this streamlined way, without all the additives and items that made you hyperactive and crazy-alert the way that sugar does. However, if you've been closely following the 8WTW plan, your body is now one big furnace of fat-burning fun!

Over the next 5 weeks you're going to notice some amazing changes, because your body is learning to work properly again. It's incredibly important that you treat your body with respect, and don't deny it the nutrients that it requires. And that means eating the ingredients that are added to The List each week. The reboot that you're doing at the moment is showing your body how to utilise the food you eat in a more efficient manner, to ensure better hair, skin, energy, and a better-functioning body all round. It's one step at a time. Just like when you're building a house, you have to get the foundations right before you can start building up.

TIP: IT'S IMPORTANT TO REMEMBER THAT THIS TRANSFORMATION ISN'T ABOUT WEIGHT LOSS. IT'S ABOUT AN ENTIRE REBOOT OF YOUR METABOLISM, WHICH MEANS FAT LOSS – AND THAT'S COMPLETELY DIFFERENT.

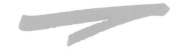

SO KEEP ON KEEPING ON, AND LET'S SHOW WEEK 4 WHO'S BOSS!

THE LIST: *WEEK 4 WEEKEND*

We gradually add foods back in to the program, so that by the end of the 8 weeks, your daily plan is back to a good balance of the items you need to make sure your body is fuelled the right way. The main thing to remember this weekend is that it isn't your last weekend ever, nor your last meal, so try not to overeat or go crazy. You've spent the past 3 weeks learning and appreciating portion control, so really put that into practice this weekend.

GRAINS (OR CORN)

On either Saturday or Sunday, eat one portion of grains or corn chosen from the list below. You can eat it at any time of the day, but just once, and just one serving size.

♀ **A serving is ½ cup of cooked grains or corn**

♂ **A serving is ⅔ cup of cooked grains or corn (or 1 cup if you are over 183 cm/6 ft tall)**

+ Brown rice
+ Buckwheat
+ Couscous (any kind)
+ Gluten-free pasta (rice or quinoa pasta)
+ Lentils
+ Oats
+ Quinoa
+ Wild rice
+ Corn (fresh)

FRUIT

On either Saturday or Sunday (not the day you have a serving of grains), choose a piece of fresh fruit to eat from the list on page 28. It must be a serving of fresh fruit – not sugared, not tinned, not stewed and not baked into something else. Banana bread does not count!

Do you absolutely have to eat this fruit? As discussed in previous weeks, it really is highly recommended that you do.

YOU WILL LOVE BEING IN CONTROL OF YOUR DIET, AND LOVE THE RESULTS. YOU'VE GOT THIS!

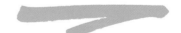

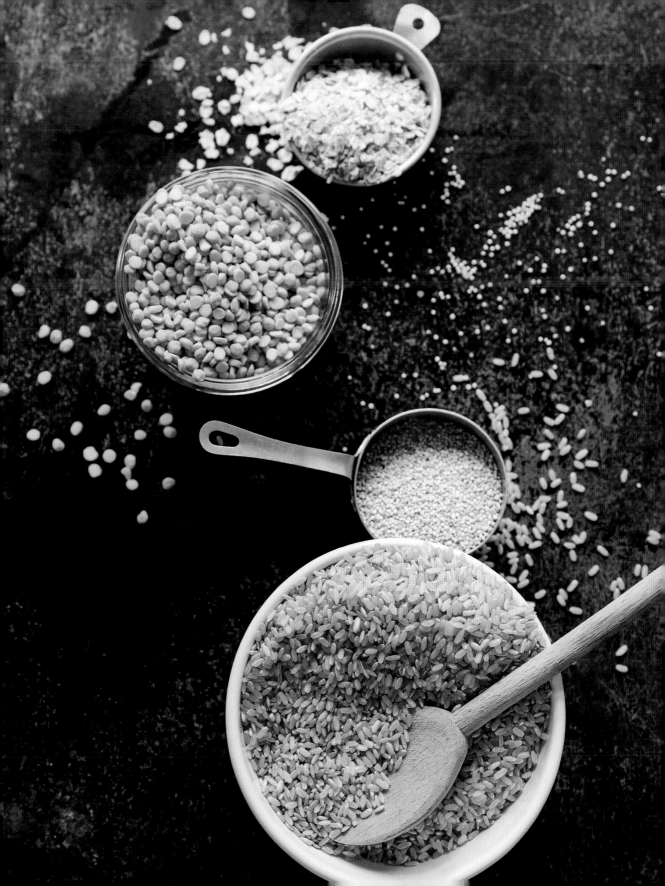

WEEK 8

WEEK 7

WEEK 6

WEEK 5

SMASHING IT!

WEEK 4

WEEK 3

WEEK 2

WEEK 1

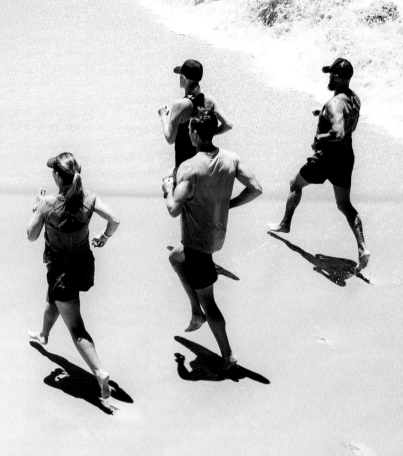

TRANSFORMATION STORIES
PATRICK'S STORY

Name: Patrick Dooley

Age: 41

Occupation: IT Manager

When did you complete the 8WTW program? September 2015

What motivated you to undertake this program?
I was convinced to give it a go over a few beers with a mate who had recently completed it and achieved seriously impressive results.

What goals did you set for yourself?
To feel good, set a good example for my kids, become a better runner, and drop years of previously unshakable body fat.

Did you meet those goals?
Absolutely. Not only those goals, but many more goals I wasn't expecting to meet and exceed.

Which aspect of the program did you find the most challenging?
The diet. Cutting out carbohydrates for the first couple of weeks and experiencing my body switch from burning those carbs for fuel to burning fat for the first time was hard. But after that, things seemed to switch, and I started experiencing considerable amounts of alertness and energy. That made it easier to stick with it.

Which week was the hardest for you? Why?
Week 1 – Day 4. This was the day my sugar cravings kicked the bucket, but not without putting up a good fight first.

Favourite exercise from the workouts?
Push-ups. I used to dislike them and burn out quickly, but through a little practice they became something I really enjoyed doing.

Which exercise did you dread the most?
Grunts (a structured burpee). Grunts can reduce most, including myself, to a gasping wreck in a short space of time, which also makes them one of the best DARC exercises in my view.

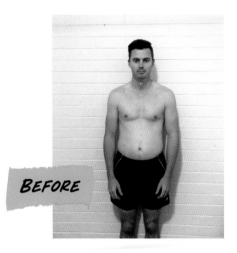

BEFORE

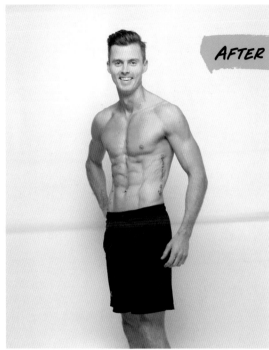

AFTER

Did you discover any new favourite foods?

Bok choy became a new favourite (it's great in a stir-fry with fresh white fish and a splash of soy sauce), and the natural taste of all fresh produce became something I loved once my tastebuds had adjusted to my healthier diet.

How did you stay motivated on hard days?

Having seen how effective the program was from friends who had completed it , I knew it would work if I just stuck to the plan. Regular group emails from Emilie, and talking to others who were doing the challenge also kept me in the right frame of mind. This helped to replace the negative thinking with positive thoughts, and shut down the excuses that can get in the way of achieving results.

What is your top tip for someone just starting?

Don't overthink things or try to rationalise the guidance provided. Trust the coaches, trust the process, and trust yourself. You can and will achieve the results you're after if you stay the course. Do it!

THE NATURAL TASTE OF ALL FRESH PRODUCE BECAME SOMETHING I LOVED ONCE MY TASTEBUDS HAD ADJUSTED TO MY HEALTHIER DIET.

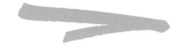

WELCOME TO WEEK 5

As you begin Week 5, you will start to notice bigger changes in your fitness, your willpower and how your clothes fit. If you have lost motivation, this is the time to compare yourself with the measurements and photos you took in Week 1. It's also a good idea to revisit your goals and remember your reasons for starting this transformation in the first place.

The grains you ate over the weekend, as well as the piece of fruit, will have your metabolism firing. And, as long as you stuck to the amounts suggested, you should be full of energy now – almost bouncing off the walls! Exercising would have been a blast this morning. You will also have noticed that you're looking a little more toned today, and that's great. It means you're heading in the right direction.

Remember not to be too hard on yourself. Be kind and give your body time to register the changes it's going through. We're going to pick up some speed again over the next couple of weeks with the physical changes, and all you need to do is follow the program and keep your eyes on the prize. And that prize is a brand-new you.

By this stage you might be asking yourself, when can I get back to eating normally? Or maybe a friend or a family member has asked you this question. The answer is, 'What is normal?' Normal to some might be a bottle or a glass of wine every night, chocolate biscuits in the afternoon or take-away for dinner. But normal to others is taking care of their body, fuelling it with foods that will keep their brain on task throughout the day, and keeping their body working and looking the way they want it to.

Habits are very easy to get hold of – both the good ones and the bad ones. If you take into account the best habit you've made over the last 5 weeks, for example, increasing your water intake, then you've made progress towards a new, healthier you.

Other habits might be preparing your lunch in advance, so that you don't get caught having to grab a quick sushi roll or two, or being able to say 'just one' at your Friday night work drinks. It's never just about the food – transformations involve the mind, body and soul. Following the 8WTW program is a way for you to work out your inner strength as well as your physical strength, using good habits to make healthy choices part of your second nature.

While some people may see these 8 weeks as a 'quick fix', we definitely don't see it that way. We are helping you to build or rebuild the foundations of a healthy plate, as well as an understanding of what fuels your body. We want you to know what makes you feel good, feel strong and, most of all, feel like the person you want to be looking back at you in the mirror.

TIP: AS YOU KICK OFF WEEK 5, STICK TO THE PROGRAM AS CLOSELY AS YOU CAN. GET YOUR WORKOUTS OR SWEAT SESSIONS IN, AND DON'T FORGET TO DRINK LOTS OF WATER. WATER IS THE MAGICAL INGREDIENT THAT WILL KEEP YOUR METABOLISM MOVING AT THE RATE WE NEED IT TO.

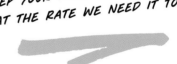

THE LIST: _WEEKS 5 & 6_

If you're a fructose-lover, it's your time to shine – we're going to start adding fruit back into your regular diet. We all have our favourite fruits. I love bananas when it comes to endurance training, and they're one of my favourite sources of carbs on race days, but I rarely eat them. I live for raspberries and blueberries – they're my daily go-to fruit. A handful of blueberries and I'm in heaven!

FRUIT

♀♂ **1 serving (shown after the item) of fresh fruit (not dried or tinned) every second day (e.g. on Monday, Wednesday, Friday and Sunday)**

Your best bet for your serving of fruit in the 8WTW program is to choose from the fruits listed here. They are listed in ascending order of sugar content, so the best choices are at the top of the list, and the ones that are higher in sugar are towards the bottom of the list.

+ Blackberries (½ cup)
+ Cranberries (½ cup)
+ Raspberries (½ cup)
+ Blueberries (½ cup)
+ Apples (1 medium)
+ Apricots (2 small)

Then you have:

+ Watermelon (1 slice)
+ Honeydew melon (1 slice)
+ Peaches (1 small)
+ Nectarines (1 small)
+ Strawberries (½ cup)

The following are a little higher in sugar, so require a smaller serving size:

+ Bananas (1 medium)
+ Grapes (1 cup) TIP: try these frozen!
+ Cherries (1 cup)
+ Mandarins (1 small)
+ Mango (1 cup)

TIP: AS WITH OTHER FOODS, THE BUILDING BLOCKS ARE SO IMPORTANT. WE'RE STILL ADDING FOODS IN A WAY THAT WILL ENSURE YOUR METABOLISM AND BODY KNOW HOW TO USE THEM, AND THAT IT DOESN'T GET OVERWHELMED BY AN INFLUX OF SIMPLE CARBS AND SIMPLE SUGARS.

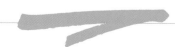

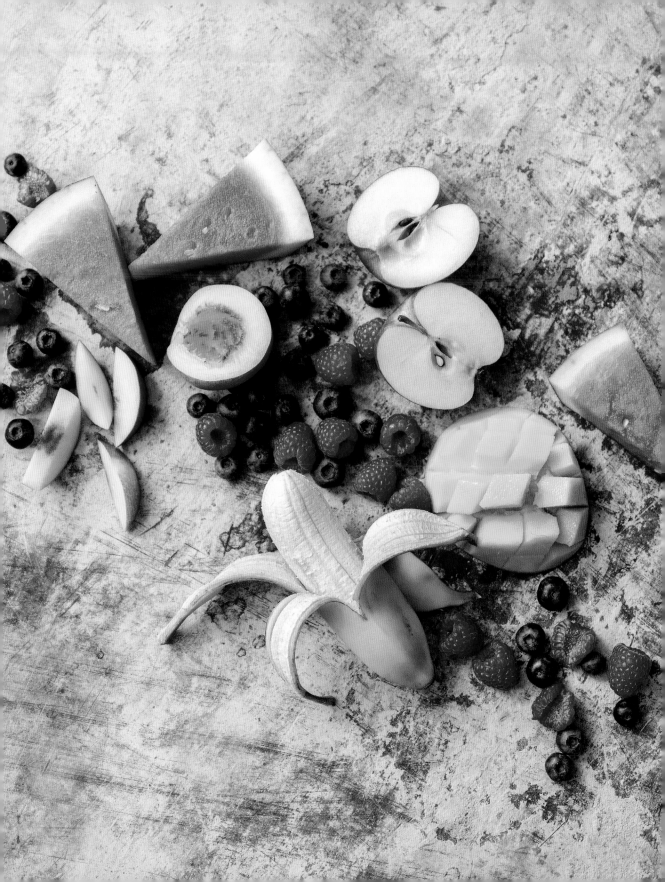

WEEK 8

WEEK 7

WEEK 6

WORK FOR IT!

~~WEEK 5~~

~~WEEK 4~~

~~WEEK 3~~

~~WEEK 2~~

~~WEEK 1~~

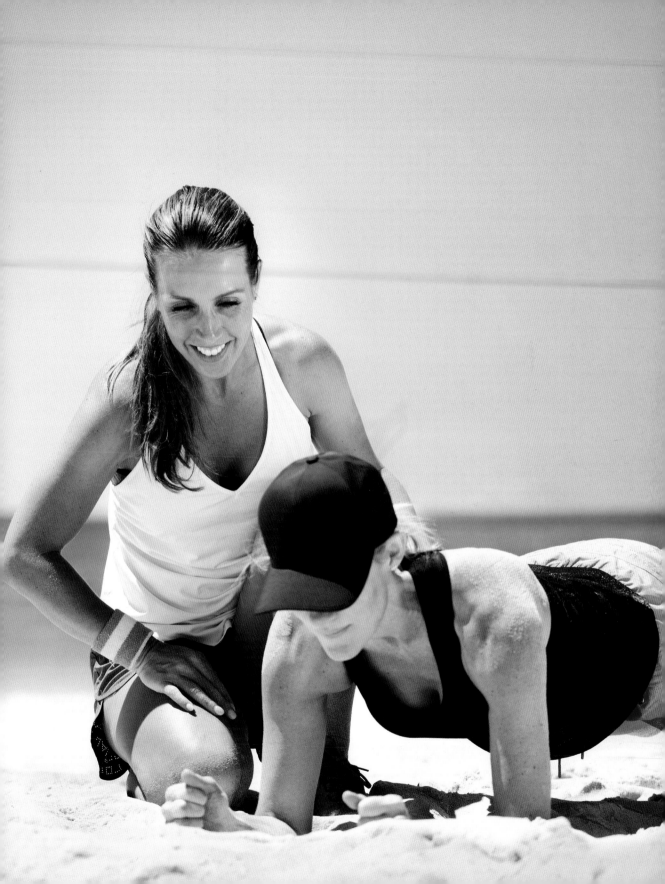

TRANSFORMATION STORIES
CONNIE'S STORY

Name: Connie Giaquinto

Age: 37

Occupation: Self-employed entrepreneur

When did you complete the 8WTW program? The first time was 2014 (I've done it 8 times, and completed it successfully 4 times!)

What motivated you to undertake this program?
I felt uncomfortable in my skin and I wanted to be fit, fast and strong.

What goals did you set for yourself?
To finish and stay true to myself.

Did you meet those goals?
100% – that's why I'm where I am today.

Which aspect of the program did you find the most challenging?
I didn't find it challenging in any one particular aspect as I was completely committed to it.

Which week was the hardest for you? Why?
I've completed the course a few times now, and each time I do it, it's the first week that's the hardest. It's not that I'm hungry it's just that my body is craving the elements of my diet that I've just cut out. If you complete the first week, you'll be OK.

Favourite exercise from the workouts?
Well that's hard cause I love everything, especially because when I first started out, I wasn't able to complete a circuit, but now I can do two in a row.

Which exercise did you dread the most?
Well, I don't really dread any. But my least favourite is push-ups – I feel they can sometimes defeat me.

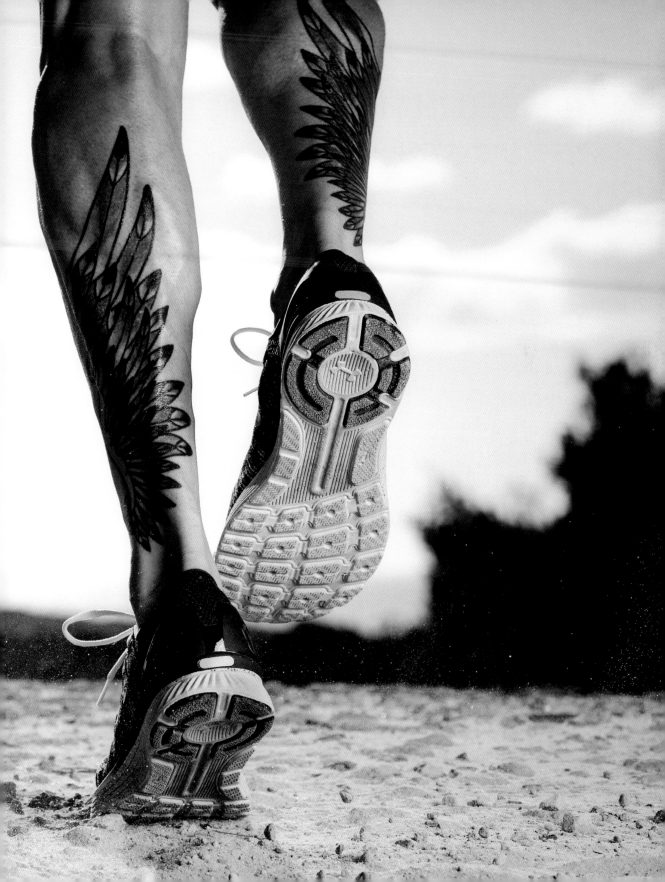

TRANSFORMATION STORIES
DUSTIN'S STORY

Name: Dustin Beasley

Age: 36

Occupation: United States Coast Guard

When did you complete the 8WTW program? My first time was September 2014.

What motivated you to undertake this program?
My original goal was to get in shape for an obstacle race. Em and Chief were incredibly supportive and set me up for success.

What goals did you set for yourself?
I wanted to lose at least 20 pounds (9 kilograms) and not get winded going up the stairs.

Did you meet those goals?
I did meet my goals. I didn't realise how bad I felt until I felt good. I wanted to feel comfortable in my own skin and not get winded going up a flight of stairs. I definitely achieved that.

Which aspect of the program did you find the most challenging?
The hardest thing was the cardio. I was in horrible shape before the challenge.

Which week was the hardest for you? Why?
The first week. It was the hardest because I wasn't active at all before I started.

Favourite exercise from the workouts?
I love the variety of push-ups! Diamond, badger and shoulder push-ups, just to name a few.

Which exercise did you dread the most?
FROGS!! I really just hate them.

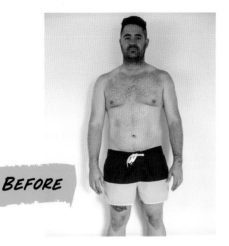

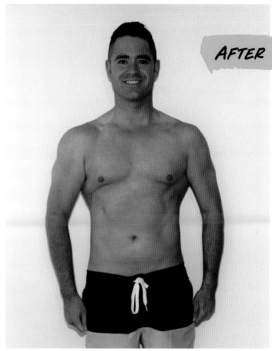

Did you discover any new favourite foods?

I love over-easy eggs served on top of a beef patty with spinach and low-fat cream cheese. I'll add bacon if I'm feeling feisty.

How did you stay motivated on hard days?

Working out consistently is good for my mental health. I was diagnosed with PTSD and Em and Chief have helped me with more than just the workouts.

What is your top tip for someone just starting?

My top tip is to support other people! I'm very active in the Facebook group – posting pictures of food, my workouts and anything inspiring. Find someone who needs encouragement and smother them with it.

I DIDN'T REALISE HOW BAD I FELT UNTIL I FELT GOOD. I WANTED TO FEEL COMFORTABLE IN MY OWN SKIN AND NOT GET WINDED GOING UP A FLIGHT OF STAIRS. I DEFINITELY ACHIEVED THAT.

WELCOME TO WEEK 7

Not long now – just a couple of weeks before you can say, 'I did it!'. Every week in the program is important, but this week is *really* important. As we head towards the pointy end of the program, it's easy to be tempted to drop the ball a little more often, or start adding in foods that aren't on The List and you really aren't ready for them yet.

THE HAPPINESS TRAP

Sometimes when people see amazing results and a difference in their fitness, happiness and body shape, they start to let things slide a bit. Happiness is awesome; it's one of the best side effects of the program. After all, being happy with yourself – both inside and out – is ultimately what 8WTW is all about. But while some people are emotional eaters and eat the wrong things when they feel down, many people also go the other way. When you're happy, you can slip up just as easily.

This is what I mean when I say that the program isn't all about the food. We all need to find that happy place in our minds, where food isn't the reward. But we definitely want you to harvest your happiness. So instead of making your reward a go-to food – whether it's a 'good' food or a 'bad' food in your mind – try rewarding yourself with something else.

Consider buying yourself some new clothes (you'll want them after all the weight you've lost!), going to the movies, getting a manicure or catching up with your favourite people. Make sure it's something that you wouldn't usually do for yourself in the course of a typical week. Go ahead and do it – reward yourself!

The reward doesn't need to be huge, just something that helps you break the habit of seeing food as a reward. Try to stay on track, and really tackle the end of this transformation. Check on your portion sizes and make sure your daily water intake is really on track.

PORTION CONTROL

Let's talk about portion control and how important it is. Hold up your hand, out in front of you. Now close your hand into a loose fist. Your stomach is the size of your closed hand, and stretching it out too regularly is why you might not be feeling satisfied after your meals. Over the last 6 weeks, you've trained your stomach back to its proper size. While it might stretch a bit to hold the food you're putting in it, your body is understanding how much it can hold and digest in one sitting, and how much you actually consume before you start to eat just for the sake of eating.

Some days, I am beyond hungry – I feel like I could eat the world. But instead of eating a huge lunch, I try to eat the usual size and then have a little more a few hours later. So rather than feeling full, I satisfy my hunger with my meal, but don't deny myself the opportunity to have a snack later if I get peckish again. I don't enjoy being hungry and I love food, so I make it work in a way that suits me and ensures that I don't have so much lunch that I need to have a sleep afterwards.

If you're hungry after you've eaten, have a think about why. Did you eat too fast? Was the meal or snack that you ate something that your body will use as fuel, or was it a bit junky? Was it tasty? There's no point in eating something that you don't like, because your mind won't be satisfied. One of the best snacks I find is anything from The Protein Bread Co. They make super-low-carb bread, muffin, pancake and pizza mixes that you've probably discovered during the last 6 weeks. My go-to is soft-boiled eggs smashed with feta or avocado on a piece of Protein Bread Co. toast. I have to stop myself going through a few slices because it tastes

so amazing! Other snacks can be as simple as a handful of fresh berries or natural almonds, a home-made protein shake or a smaller portion of left-over breakfast, lunch or dinner.

GO BACK THROUGH THE RECIPES FROM PREVIOUS WEEKS, AND HIGHLIGHT SOME OF YOUR FAVOURITE MEALS AND SNACKS. YOU MIGHT HAVE FORGOTTEN ABOUT SOME OF THEM BECAUSE YOU'VE BEEN BUSY TRYING NEW RECIPES AND INGREDIENTS. TAKE A LOOK AT ANYTHING YOU HAVEN'T TRIED YET - YOU NEVER KNOW, YOU MIGHT NOW LIKE SOME OF THE RECIPES YOU SKIPPED OVER A FEW WEEKS AGO.

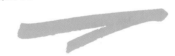

THE LIST: *WEEKS 7 & 8*

After all those practice weekends of monitoring your portion sizes and different grains, here's where we start to use your new skills more regularly.

GRAINS

On Tuesdays, Thursdays and Saturdays, eat one portion of grains, chosen from the list below.

 A serving is ½ cup of cooked grains

 A serving is ⅔ cup of cooked grains (or 1 cup if you're over 183 cm/6 ft tall)

+ Brown rice
+ Buckwheat
+ Couscous (any kind)
+ Gluten-free pasta (rice or quinoa pasta)
+ Lentils
+ Oats
+ Quinoa
+ Wild rice

Alternatively, you may choose to eat the same size portion of sweet potato or fresh corn.

IMPORTANT

You will get the best results if you ease grains back into your diet, which is why we start by having them only every second day to begin with. Remember to keep a good eye on your portion sizes.

Once you have completed Week 8, you can organise how often you want these items, and whether you feel like you need them every day, every second day, or even just on the weekends. It's really up to you, and knowing how your body works with the foods you're eating now.

Try to start your week clean every Monday. Drink 2–3 litres (70–105 fl oz/8–12 cups) of water, eat lots of your compulsory greens, colourful vegies and clean protein, such as fish, chicken and lean meats.

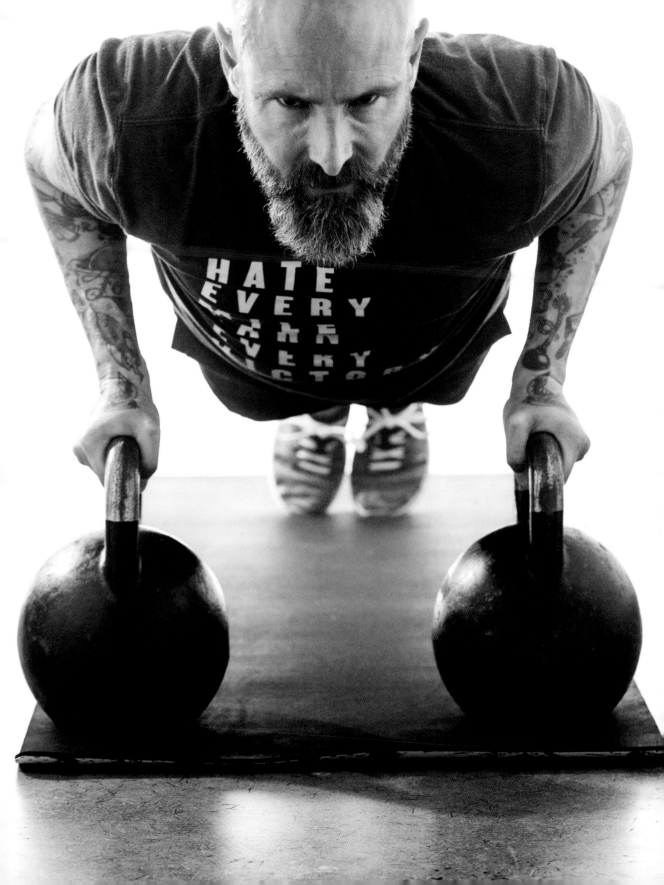

WEEK 8

SMASH YOUR GOAL!

WEEK 7

WEEK 6

WEEK 5

WEEK 4

WEEK 3

WEEK 2

WEEK 1

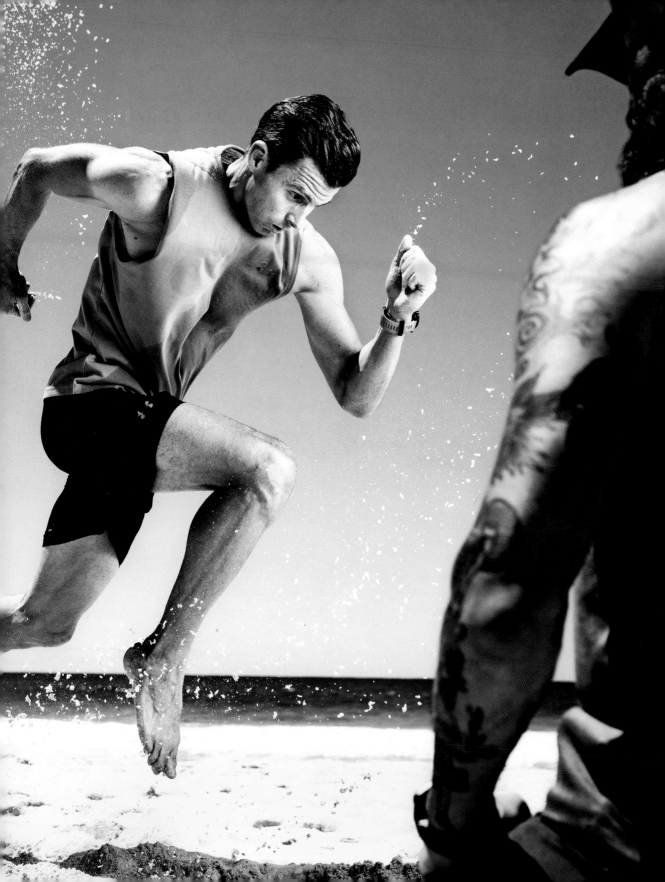

TRANSFORMATION STORIES
ROSIE'S STORY

Name: Rosie Alys Hames (AKA Em's little sister!)
Age: 31
Occupation: Full-time mum
When did you complete the 8WTW program? 2015

What motivated you to undertake this program?
I had just had my first child and I wanted to feel like myself again. I'm sure most mothers will agree that once you've had a child or two, your body is no longer yours completely. I missed it, and I missed the control – I wanted to be in charge of my own shape.

What goals did you set for yourself?
To eat according to the plan, to try as hard as I could in the workouts and to make my sister proud.

Did you meet those goals?
Yes, and exceeded them! I was back int my pre-pregnancy clothing within 2 months.

Which aspect of the program did you find the most challenging?
Cutting out the foods I'd become used to with my pregnancy cravings.

Which week was the hardest for you? Why?
Definitely week 1! I was tired and cranky and just wanted to be able to grab something easy and fast to eat.

Favourite exercise from the workouts?
Definitely pull-ups. I don't know why, but I really like them!

Which exercise did you dread the most?
Ab work! I was weakest there.

Did you discover any new favourite foods?
Not just favourite foods, but I discovered that my tastebuds changed over the 8 weeks. What I thought of as 'diet food' in the beginning is now a staple in my house, and the kids love munching on carrot sticks and hummus!

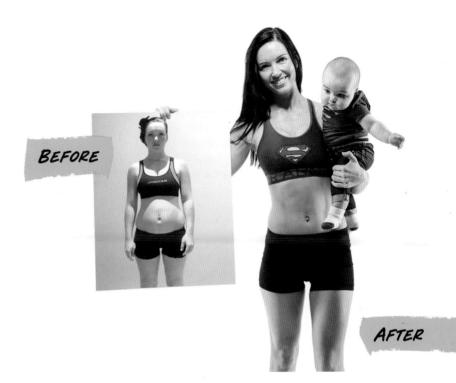

BEFORE

AFTER

How did you stay motivated on hard days?

I would talk to my sister, Em, remind myself of how and why I was doing it, and then take another look at my favourite pair of jeans – I wanted to wear them again!

What is your top tip for someone just starting?

Don't put it off – just dive right in. It's always tough to get started but with the right attitude you can achieve anything.

WHAT I THOUGHT OF AS 'DIET FOOD' IN THE BEGINNING IS NOW A STAPLE IN MY HOUSE, AND THE KIDS LOVE MUNCHING ON CARROT STICKS AND HUMMUS!

WELCOME TO WEEK 8

We're here, and I'm so impressed with how far you've come. Can you believe you're heading into the final week of your transformation? I really hope that this program (or at least some of it) has become second nature to you, and that you feel completely amazing. Seriously – how good do you feel?

If you haven't met your goals yet, don't worry. The simple fact is that you have now educated yourself in a way that means you can stick to a healthier way of eating and training if you want to. Those habits that you didn't think would have stuck have done so, otherwise you wouldn't still be here in Week 8. All you need to do is keep moving forward. Use all the tools you've developed in the last 8 weeks to continue making progress. It's all about taking one step at a time.

This transformation wasn't ever just about food. It has always been about three things:

[1] Changing your body
[2] Changing your way of thinking
[3] Changing the way you move and train

Remember that a 'clean' week of drinking water and eating fresh food can do wonders for your skin, mind and body. Try to really make sure that you get to the end of this week and make the most of all the hard work you've put in over the last 8 weeks.

LET'S GET WEEK 8 DONE!

BY THIS STAGE YOU MIGHT HAVE DIFFERENT SLEEPING PATTERNS, DIFFERENT TRAINING HOURS, EVEN NEW PASTIMES AND FAVOURITE ACTIVITIES. IT'S AMAZING WHAT A HEALTHIER OUTLOOK ON LIFE CAN DO.

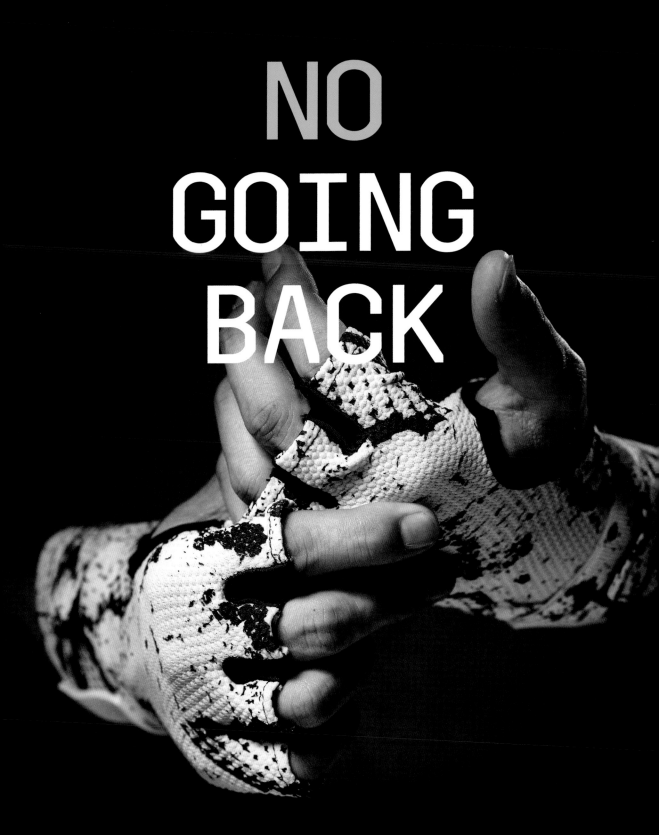

THE   RE

CIPES//

WEEK 1
RECIPES

BREAKFAST BACON BRUSCHETTA

Serves 1

½ small onion, very thinly sliced
2 tablespoons low-sodium chicken stock
salt and freshly ground black pepper
2 slices lean bacon, trimmed
1 teaspoon crushed garlic
1 tablespoon grated parmesan cheese
1 tablespoon snipped chives
1 handful baby English spinach

Heat a non-stick frying pan over medium heat. Cook the onion, stirring, until it begins to brown. Add the chicken stock, salt and pepper, reduce the heat to low and leave to simmer.

Meanwhile, fry the bacon in a separate non-stick frying pan over medium-high heat until cooked.

Arrange the bacon on a plate. Brush with the garlic and top with the hot onion. Sprinkle with the parmesan and chives, and serve with the spinach on the side. Top with a poached egg if you're really hungry.

PROTEIN PANCAKES

Serves 1

3 tablespoons low-carb Greek-style plain yoghurt
2 eggs + 1 egg white
1 scoop (30 g/1 oz) banana protein powder
1/2 teaspoon ground cinnamon
1/2 sachet sweetener

Whisk the yoghurt, eggs and egg white together in a bowl.

Combine the protein powder, cinnamon and sweetener in a separate bowl. Pour in the yoghurt mixture and whisk until smooth.

Heat a non-stick frying pan over medium heat. Pour in a ladleful of the batter and cook for 2–3 minutes or until bubbles start to appear on the surface. Turn and cook the other side until golden. Remove the pancake from the pan and keep warm while you cook the remaining batter.

These pancakes are delicious by themselves in the early weeks, but feel free to top them with a little yoghurt and a few fresh berries once fruit is back on the menu (starting on the weekend of Week 4).

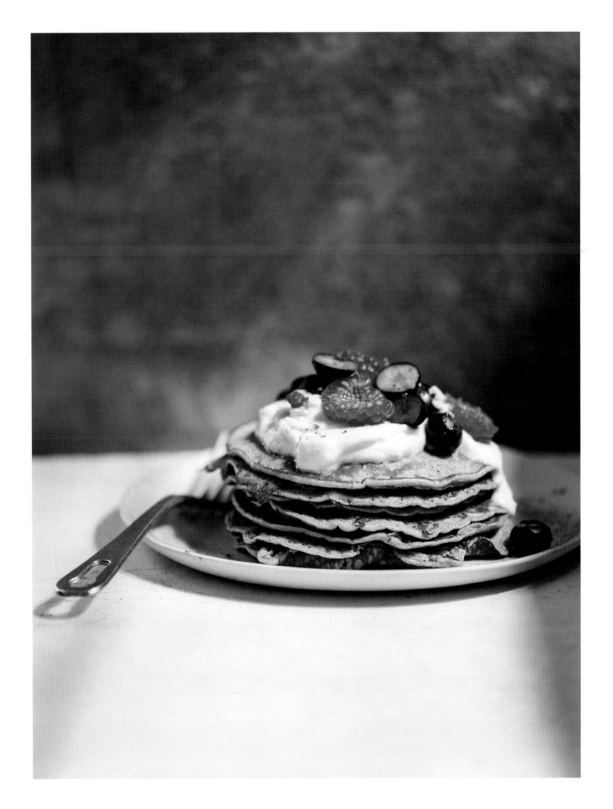

PORK LARB IN LETTUCE CUPS

Serves 4

500 g (1 lb 2 oz) lean minced (ground) pork
2 red onions, finely diced
2 cm (3/4 inch) piece fresh ginger, peeled and grated
1 fresh red chilli, thinly sliced or 1 teaspoon chilli flakes,
    plus extra for garnish
1 red or yellow capsicum (pepper), diced
2 teaspoons salt-reduced soy sauce
3 tablespoons lime juice
1 iceberg lettuce, leaves separated
low-carb plain yoghurt, to serve (optional)

Heat a wok or large non-stick frying pan over high heat. Add the
pork and cook, stirring and breaking up any lumps, for 5 minutes
or until golden. Tip out any juices. Remove the pork from the pan
and set aside.

Reheat the wok and cook the onion, ginger and chilli until fragrant
and the onion is translucent. Return the pork to the pan, add the
capsicum and mix well. Add the soy sauce and mix well, then add
the lime juice and simmer for a few minutes.

Serve the pork larb in lettuce cups, sprinkled with a little chilli or
a small dollop of yoghurt.

CRAB AND AVOCADO ROLLS »

Serves 2

170 g (5¾ oz) tin crab meat, drained
2–3 tablespoons extra-light cream cheese
2 tablespoons lime juice
salt and freshly ground black pepper
4 nori sheets
½ avocado, thinly sliced
½ Lebanese (short) cucumber, cut into thin matchsticks

Squeeze any excess liquid from the crab meat. Put the crab
meat, cream cheese, lime juice, salt and pepper in a food
processor or blender, and blend to a paste.

Place one nori sheet on a sushi mat or board. Thinly spread a
quarter of the crab mixture over the nori. Arrange a quarter
of the avocado and cucumber on top, then roll up. Repeat to
make four rolls. Enjoy as a snack or for a light lunch.

BREAKFAST CASSEROLE TO GO

Serves 4

½ onion, chopped
½ red capsicum (pepper), chopped
350 g (12 oz) lean minced (ground) pork
8 eggs, lightly beaten
1 tablespoon salt-reduced soy sauce
½ teaspoon chilli powder (optional)

Preheat the oven to 170°C (340°F).

Heat a non-stick frying pan over medium-high heat. Brown the onion, then add the capsicum and transfer to a bowl.

Add the pork to the pan and cook over medium-high heat, stirring to break up any lumps, for 5 minutes or until golden. Add to the bowl with the onion mixture.

Pour the eggs and soy sauce into an ovenproof dish. Add the chilli powder (if using). Add the pork and onion mixture and stir until well combined.

Bake for 30 minutes or until cooked through. Cut into squares and store in an airtight container in the fridge for up to 3 days.

CREAM OF ASPARAGUS SOUP

Serves 6

canola oil
1 onion, diced
1 kg (2 lb 4 oz) asparagus, cut into 5 cm (2 inch) lengths
1.5 litres (52 fl oz/6 cups) low-sodium chicken stock
salt and freshly ground black pepper
2 tablespoons low-fat sour cream

Heat a little canola oil in a large saucepan over medium heat. Sauté the onion until slightly brown.

Add the asparagus and cook for 2 minutes, then pour in the stock, and season with salt and pepper. Simmer the soup for 25–30 minutes or until the asparagus is very soft.

Allow the soup to cool slightly, then transfer to a blender. Add the sour cream and blend until smooth. Serve immediately or gently reheat if needed.

ZUCCHINI GAZPACHO WITH DICED RED CAPSICUM

Serves 6

1 low-sodium chicken stock (bouillon) cube
700 g (1 lb 9 oz) baby zucchini (courgettes), cut in half
½ teaspoon curry powder
20 g (¾ oz) chopped French shallots
salt and freshly ground black pepper
1 red capsicum (pepper), diced

Bring a large saucepan of water to the boil. Dissolve the stock cube in the boiling water. Add the zucchini and cook for 4 minutes.

Drain the zucchini, reserving 400 ml (14 fl oz) of the stock. Place the stock in the fridge for 30 minutes to cool.

Add the zucchini, curry powder and chopped shallots to a blender with the cooled stock and blend until combined. Season with salt and pepper. Return to the fridge to chill for at least 2 hours.

Divide the chilled soup between bowls and serve topped with the diced capsicum.

146

BARBECUED SALMON

Serves 2

2 salmon fillets

Marinade
2 tablespoons salt-reduced soy sauce
2 teaspoons lemon juice
½ teaspoon minced garlic
1 teaspoon grated fresh ginger
diced fresh red chilli, to taste
1 handful coriander (cilantro) leaves, roughly chopped
1 lemongrass stem, pale part only, thinly sliced (optional)

To make the marinade, put the soy sauce, lemon juice, garlic, ginger, chilli, coriander and lemongrass (if using) in a bowl and mix to combine. Add the salmon and turn to coat. Leave to marinate for 10 minutes.

Preheat a barbecue for indirect cooking over high heat. Cook the salmon, skin side down, for 10–12 minutes or until done to your liking. Do not overcook the salmon or it will dry out. Serve hot.

NOTE: BARBECUING GIVES THE SALMON A LOVELY BUTTERY TEXTURE. SERVE WITH BABY ENGLISH SPINACH.

HOT AND SOUR BEEF SOUP WITH LIME

Serves 4

2.5 litres (87 fl oz/10 cups) low-sodium beef stock

2 lemongrass stems, pale parts only, halved

3 garlic cloves, halved

2.5 cm (1 inch) piece fresh ginger, sliced

1 small fresh red chilli, seeded and finely chopped, plus extra for garnish

90 g (3¼ oz/1 bunch) coriander (cilantro), leaves and stems separated, leaves chopped

2 strips lime zest

2 star anise

4 spring onions (scallions), thinly sliced on the diagonal

500 g (1 lb 2 oz) fillet or rump steak, trimmed

1 tablespoon salt-reduced soy sauce

2 tablespoons lime juice

freshly ground black pepper

lime wedges, to serve

Put the stock, lemongrass, garlic, ginger, chilli, coriander stems, lime zest, star anise and half the spring onion in a large saucepan. Bring to the boil over a high heat, then reduce the heat and simmer, covered, for 25 minutes. Strain the stock, discarding the solids, then return the stock to the pan.

Heat a chargrill or non-stick frying pan over high heat. Sear the steak on both sides until brown on the outside but quite rare in the centre. (Feel free to cook a little more if you prefer your meat more well done.)

Reheat the soup over medium heat. Add the soy sauce and lime juice, to taste, and season with pepper. Add most of the remaining spring onion and most of the coriander leaves.

Thinly slice the beef across the grain. Divide among four bowls and pour the hot soup over the top. Garnish with chilli, some reserved spring onion and coriander leaves and serve with lime wedges.

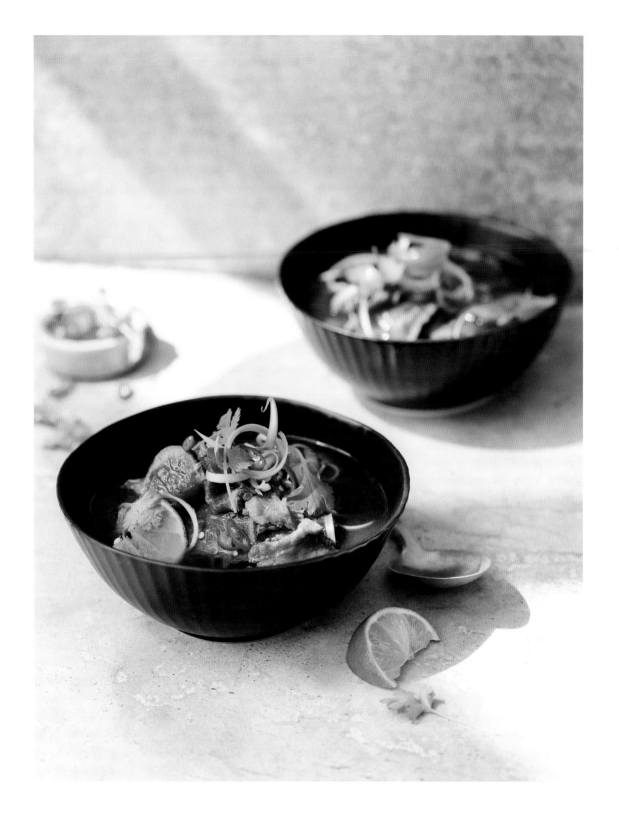

CARBONARA

Serves 1

½ small onion, diced
2 slices lean bacon, trimmed and diced
30 g (1 oz) cooked lean chicken, diced
1 garlic clove, crushed
125 g (4½ oz) konjac fettuccine noodles
1 egg
1 tablespoon grated parmesan cheese
freshly ground black pepper, to taste

Heat a non-stick frying pan over medium heat. Cook the onion, bacon and chicken for 5 minutes or until the onion and bacon are cooked and the chicken is heated through. Stir in the garlic.

Add the noodles, then stir in the egg, parmesan and pepper and cook until the noodles are hot and the egg has created a silky sauce.

OVEN-COOKED BARRAMUNDI

Serves 4

600 g (1 lb 5 oz) barramundi (see Note)
juice of ½ lemon or 3 tablespoons red wine vinegar
½ teaspoon salt
½ teaspoon ground black pepper
1 tablespoon dried coriander (cilantro)
1 tablespoon dried rosemary
1 tablespoon dried thyme
400 g (14 oz) shredded iceberg lettuce
100 g (3½ oz) low-fat cottage cheese

Preheat the oven to 180°C (350°F). Line a large, deep roasting tin with foil. Place the barramundi in the tin, skin side down. Drizzle with the lemon juice or vinegar and sprinkle with the salt, pepper and dried herbs. Cover the tin with foil and bake the barramundi for 35 minutes or until the flesh flakes apart easily when tested.

Remove the skin from the barramundi. Divide the shredded lettuce and fish among four plates. Serve topped with the cottage cheese.

NOTE: USE A WHOLE BARRAMUNDI FILLET OR FOUR 150 G (5½ OZ) PIECES.

BARBECUED CHILLI OCTOPUS WITH GARLIC YOGHURT

Serves 2

500 g (1 lb 2 oz) baby octopus, cleaned
2 garlic cloves, thinly sliced
3 small fresh red chillies, seeded and finely chopped
1½ teaspoons chopped oregano or basil
dill sprigs, to serve

Garlic yoghurt
200 g (7 oz) low-fat Greek-style plain yoghurt
1 garlic clove, crushed
sea salt flakes

Halve the octopus heads and quarter the tentacles. Place in a heatproof bowl and cover with boiling water. Leave to stand for 1–2 minutes, then drain.

Combine the sliced garlic, chilli and oregano or basil in another bowl. Add the octopus pieces, cover and marinate for at least 30 minutes.

To make the garlic yoghurt, combine the yoghurt, crushed garlic and salt, to taste. Refrigerate until needed.

Preheat a barbecue or chargrill plate to high. Remove the octopus from the marinade and cook, turning occasionally, for 2–5 minutes or until slightly charred.

Pile the octopus onto a platter, garnish with dill sprigs and serve with the garlic yoghurt on the side.

NOTE: YOU CAN ALSO USE CALAMARI, SQUID OR CUTTLEFISH, CUT INTO LARGE STRIPS, OR LARGE PRAWNS (SHRIMP), OMITTING THE BOILING WATER STEP.

FISH WITH HERBS

Serves 2

2 firm white fish fillets
salt and freshly ground black pepper
mixed fresh herbs, such as basil, parsley, oregano and dill

Cut the fish into bite-sized chunks and place in a bowl. Season with salt and pepper.

Mix the herbs together and chop finely. Sprinkle the herbs over the fish and toss to coat.

Heat a non-stick frying pan over medium heat. Add the fish pieces and cook, turning, for 5-10 minutes or until golden and just cooked through. Serve immediately.

COMBINATION RISSOLES »

Serves 4

1 zucchini (courgette), roughly chopped
1 onion, roughly chopped
300 g (10½ oz) lean minced (ground) chicken
300 g (10½ oz) lean minced (ground) pork
200 g (7 oz) peeled raw prawns (shrimp), finely diced
2 eggs
½ teaspoon ancho chilli
½ teaspoon smoked chipotle chilli
2 garlic cloves, crushed
6 basil leaves, finely chopped or 2 teaspoons dried basil
salt-reduced soy sauce, to serve

Preheat the oven to 200°C (400°F). Line a baking tray with baking paper.

Put the zucchini and onion in a food processor and chop until very fine. Transfer to a large bowl and add the chicken, pork, prawns, eggs, chillies, garlic and basil. Mix until well combined.

Take heaped tablespoons of the mixture and form it into balls. Place on the baking tray and bake for 20 minutes or until golden brown. Serve the rissoles hot or cold with a splash of soy sauce.

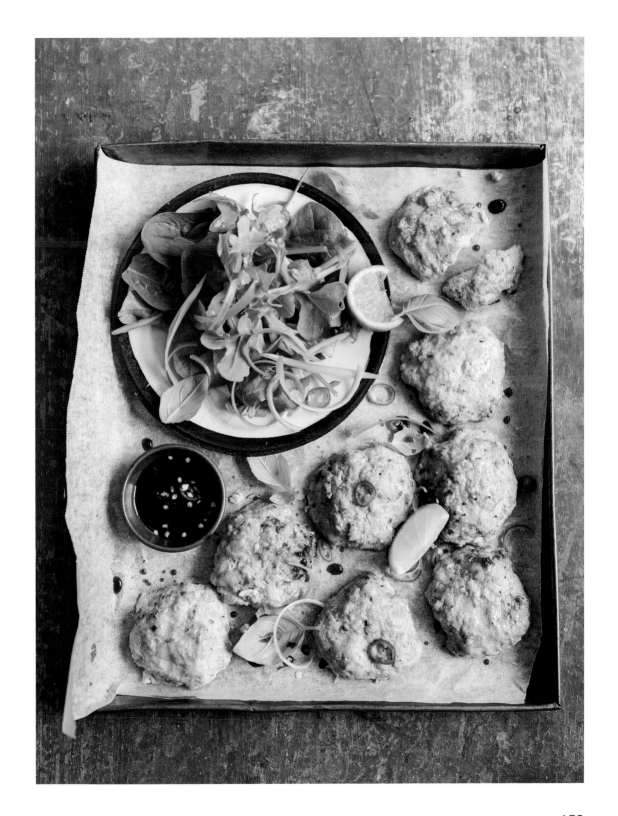

INFERNO BURRITO

Serves 2

2 skinless chicken breast fillets, cut into strips
1/4 onion, sliced
1 garlic clove, crushed
1 teaspoon chilli powder, or to taste
1 teaspoon ground cumin
1 teaspoon paprika
1 teaspoon ground coriander
1/2 teaspoon ground cinnamon
1/2 teaspoon cayenne pepper
1 egg + 250 ml (9 fl oz) egg whites
extra-light sour cream, to serve
coriander (cilantro) leaves, to serve (optional)

Heat a non-stick frying pan over medium heat. Brown the
chicken, then add the onion and garlic and cook until the onion
is translucent. Add the spices and 125 ml (4 fl oz/1/2 cup) water.
Gently simmer until the chicken is cooked through and the
water has evaporated. Remove from the heat.

Whisk the egg and egg whites together in a bowl. Pour into a
non-stick frying pan over medium-high heat and cook until
almost set. Arrange the chicken in the centre and add a little sour
cream. Fold up the ends, then fold in the sides and cut in half.
Serve immediately, sprinkled with coriander.

ASIAN-STYLE MUSSELS »

Serves 2-3

1 kg (2 lb 4 oz) mussels
1/2 red onion, sliced
1 garlic clove, sliced
1 teaspoon chilli flakes
grated zest and juice of 1 lemon
2 tablespoons salt-reduced soy sauce
1 handful roughly chopped coriander (cilantro),
    plus extra leaves to serve

Discard any mussels that are open and don't close when tapped
on the bench. Scrub the mussel shells until clean, remove the
beards and place in a colander to drain.

Put the onion, garlic, chilli flakes and lemon zest in a large
saucepan. Pour in half the lemon juice and cook over medium
heat until the onion is translucent. Add the mussels, soy sauce,
chopped coriander and remaining lemon juice. Cover and cook
for 5-7 minutes or until the mussels open (discard any that
don't open).

Transfer the mussels to a large serving bowl. Pour over the
cooking juices and garnish with coriander leaves.

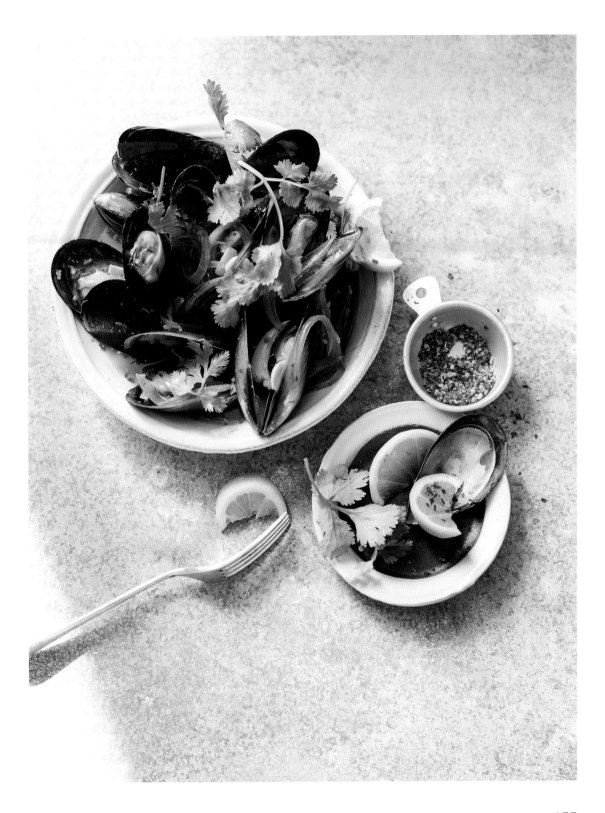

MOCHA SHAKE »
Serves 1

250 ml (9 fl oz/1 cup) skim or non-fat milk or
    unsweetened almond milk
2 teaspoons fat-free sugar-free hot chocolate mix
1 instant coffee sachet or 1 teaspoon instant coffee
1 sachet of sweetener
135 g (4¾ oz/1 cup) ice cubes

Pour the milk into a high-powered blender. Add the hot chocolate
mix, coffee, sweetener and ice cubes. Blend until smooth, then
serve immediately.

PROTEIN ICE CREAM »
Serves 2

60 g (2 oz) extra-light ricotta cheese
1 teaspoon fat-free Greek-style plain yoghurt
1 scoop (30 g/1 oz) vanilla protein powder
2 drops natural vanilla extract

Put the ricotta, yoghurt, protein powder and vanilla in a bowl.
Mix until well combined. Transfer to a freezer-proof container
and freeze for 30 minutes or until firm.

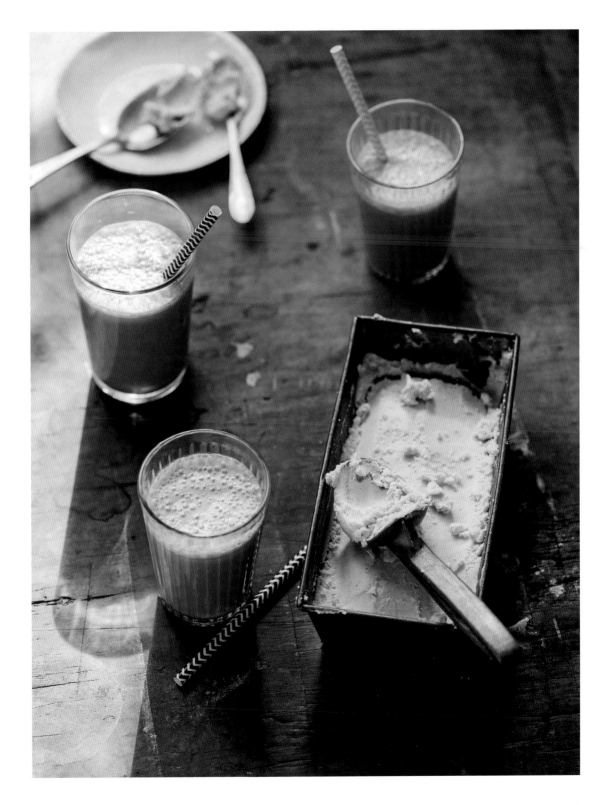

WEEK 3
RECIPES

MEXICAN BREAKFAST

Serves 2

1 tomato, diced
¼ red onion, diced
¼ brown onion, diced
2 handfuls finely chopped parsley
2 teaspoons minced garlic
4 shakes of Tabasco sauce
2 tablespoons lime juice
salt and freshly ground black pepper
4 large eggs

Combine the tomato, onions and parsley in a bowl.

In a separate bowl, mix the garlic and Tabasco well. Pour into the tomato mixture and mix until combined. Sprinkle the lime juice over the top and season with salt and pepper. Set aside.

Heat a non-stick frying pan over medium heat. Lightly beat the eggs until combined. Pour into the hot pan and cook, gently stirring until the eggs are just set.

Divide the scrambled egg between two bowls and spoon the tomato salsa on top. Serve immediately.

B2B FRITTERS

Serves 4

2–3 slices lean bacon, trimmed
2 zucchini (courgettes)
4 eggs, lightly beaten
1 handful shredded basil
chilli flakes, to taste
salt and freshly ground black pepper
lime wedges, for squeezing

Avo smash (optional)
¼ avocado
2 cherry tomatoes, diced
1 small handful shredded basil
lime wedges, for squeezing
salt and freshly ground black pepper

To make the avo smash, roughly mash the avocado in a bowl. Add the diced tomatoes, basil and a good squeeze of lime. Sprinkle with salt and pepper and mix until just combined. Cover and refrigerate until ready to serve.

Heat a non-stick frying pan over medium–high heat. Fry the bacon until cooked and golden on both sides, then drain on paper towel. Cut into small pieces and set aside.

Grate the zucchini into a bowl and squeeze with your hands to remove the excess liquid. Stir in the eggs, basil and bacon pieces. Add the chilli flakes and season with salt and pepper, then mix well.

Heat a large non-stick frying pan over medium heat. Spoon the mixture into the pan to make four fritters. Cook, turning every 1–2 minutes to ensure even cooking, for about 8 minutes in total or until the fritters are golden and cooked through.

Serve the fritters with a squeeze of lime juice and a side of avo smash (if using).

NOTE: THESE FRITTERS ARE LOVELY TOPPED WITH A POACHED EGG. COOK THE FRITTERS IN NON-STICK EGG RINGS TO HELP THEM HOLD TOGETHER.

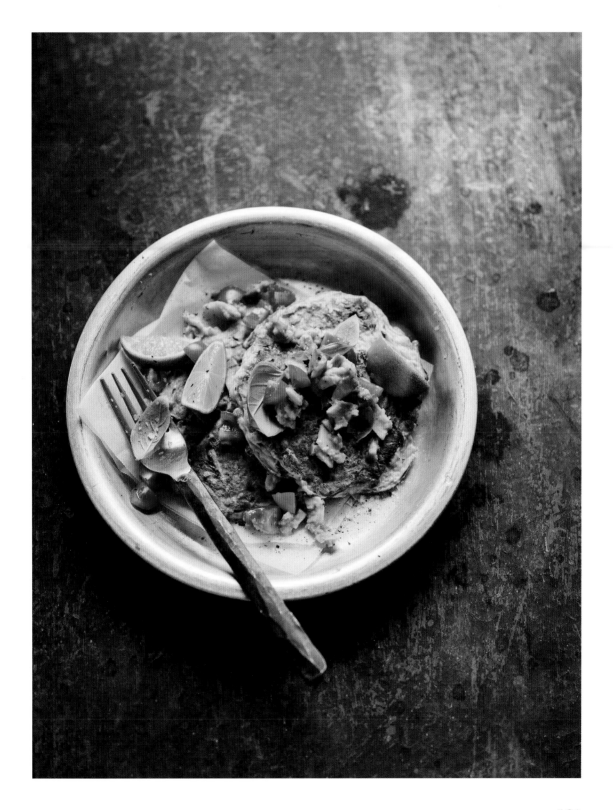

EGGPLANT LASAGNE

Serves 3-4

1 red onion, finely chopped
1 garlic clove, finely chopped
600 g (1 lb 5 oz) lean minced (ground) beef
3 tablespoons tomato paste (concentrated purée)
2 teaspoons dried basil
1 teaspoon salt
¼ teaspoon freshly ground black pepper
1 large eggplant (aubergine)

Cheese topping
300 g (10½ oz) low-fat sour cream
50 g (1¾ oz) low-fat grated cheddar cheese
60 g (2¼ oz) grated parmesan cheese
1 handful parsley, finely chopped
½ teaspoon salt
¼ teaspoon freshly ground black pepper

Heat a large non-stick frying pan over medium heat. Sauté the onion and garlic until soft. Add the beef and cook, stirring and breaking up any lumps, for 5 minutes or until browned. Stir in 125 ml (4 fl oz/½ cup water), the tomato paste, basil, salt and pepper. Bring to the boil, then reduce the heat and simmer for 10-15 minutes or until most of the water has evaporated.

Meanwhile, thinly slice the eggplant.

Preheat the oven to 200°C (400°F). Grease a 23 x 33 cm (9 x 13 inch) ovenproof dish.

To make the topping, mix the sour cream with the cheddar and most of the parmesan (reserve 1-2 tablespoons for sprinkling). Stir in the parsley, salt and pepper.

Layer the eggplant slices and the beef mixture in the ovenproof dish, alternating between them and finishing with a layer of eggplant. Spread the cheese topping over the eggplant and sprinkle over the reserved parmesan. Bake for 30-40 minutes or until the eggplant is cooked and the top is browned. Serve with a green salad.

NOTE: PREPARE THE BEEF AND TOMATO MIXTURE A DAY AHEAD FOR A MORE FLAVOURSOME SAUCE.

162

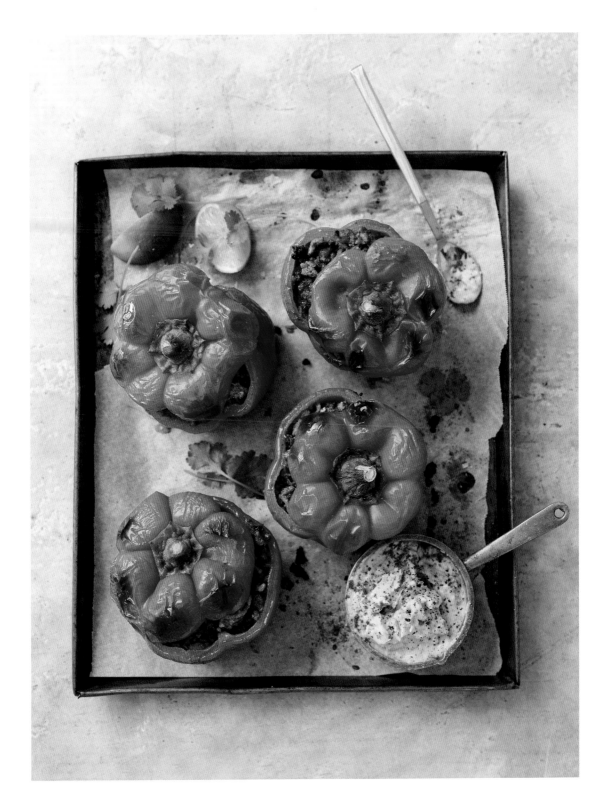

STUFFED MUSHIES

Serves 5

30 g (1 oz/½ cup) breadcrumbs made from crumbled Protein
    bread (from The Protein Bread Co.)
50 g (1¾ oz/½ cup) finely grated parmesan cheese
2 garlic cloves, crushed
2 tablespoons chopped parsley
1 tablespoon chopped mint
2 tablespoons melted coconut oil
salt and freshly ground black pepper
20 large mushrooms

Preheat the oven grill (broiler) to 200°C (400°F). Line two large
baking trays with baking paper.

Put the breadcrumbs, parmesan, garlic, parsley, mint and half
the coconut oil in a bowl. Season with salt and pepper and mix
until well combined.

Remove and discard the mushroom stems. Place the mushrooms
on the baking trays and fill with the breadcrumb mixture. Drizzle
the remaining coconut oil over the top. Bake for 20–25 minutes
or until browned. Serve hot.

NOTE: Depending on the size of your oven, you may need
to cook the mushrooms in batches, or switch the trays around
halfway through cooking.

ITALIAN CHICKEN WITH BRUSSELS SPROUTS

Serves 6

6 skinless chicken thigh fillets
12 brussels sprouts, sliced
½ red onion, sliced
2 tomatoes, diced
80 ml (2½ fl oz/⅓ cup) low-sodium chicken stock

Heat a large non-stick frying pan over medium heat. Cook
the chicken, brussels sprouts and onion until browned.

Stir in the diced tomatoes and stock. Cover and simmer
for 25 minutes, then remove the lid and simmer for another
5 minutes or until the chicken is cooked through and the
sauce has thickened. Serve immediately.

GREEN TEA FROZEN YOGHURT

Serves 2

125 ml (4 fl oz/½ cup) skim or non-fat milk
2 tablespoons green tea-leaves (see Note)
2 tablespoons sugar substitute or equivalent
200 g (7 oz/¾ cup) low-fat, low-carb Greek-style
   plain yoghurt

Combine the milk, tea and sugar substitute in a small saucepan. Heat until almost boiling, then remove from the heat and set aside to steep for 1 hour.

Strain the cooled tea mixture and stir in the yoghurt. Pour into an ice-cream maker and churn until frozen. Alternatively, pour the mixture into a shallow baking tray, cover with plastic wrap and freeze for 3 hours or until almost firm. Transfer to a food processor and blend until smooth and creamy, then return to the tray and freeze overnight. Remove from the freezer a few minutes before serving.

NOTE: USE EITHER LOOSE-LEAF GREEN TEA OR TEA BAGS.

CUCUMBER REFRESHER

Makes 1.5 litres (52 fl oz/6 cups)

1.5 litres (52 fl oz/6 cups) chilled water
1 lime
½ lemon
1 Lebanese (short) cucumber
ice cubes, to serve

Pour the chilled water into a large jug. Squeeze the lime and lemon into the water. Peel the cucumber into ribbons, straight into the water. Add the ice cubes and serve.

WEEK 4
RECIPES

SKILLET BREAKFAST

Serves 1

1 egg + 2 egg whites
30 g (1 oz) English spinach, roughly chopped
2–3 mushrooms, sliced (optional)
1 tablespoon grated low-fat cheddar cheese (optional)
15 g (1/2 oz) Protein pancake mix (from The Protein Bread Co.)

Put the egg, egg whites, spinach, mushrooms and cheese (if using) in a bowl. Add the pancake mix and whisk until combined.

Heat a non-stick frying pan over medium-low heat. Pour in the egg mixture and spread the spinach and mushrooms out around the pan. Cook for 2–3 minutes or until the base is golden, then flip and cook until golden on the other side. Watch closely as the egg whites will burn quickly. Serve immediately.

PARMESAN POACHED EGGS WITH ASPARAGUS

Serves 2

8 asparagus spears
white vinegar
4 eggs
1/2 teaspoon coconut oil
1 garlic clove, crushed
salt and freshly ground black pepper
2 teaspoons grated parmesan cheese

Blanch the asparagus spears in a saucepan of boiling water for 2 minutes, then remove and drain.

Add a splash of white vinegar to a saucepan of boiling water. Break each egg into a cup, then carefully pour into the water. Cook, without stirring, until the egg whites have set. Remove the eggs with a slotted spoon and drain on paper towel.

While the eggs are cooking, heat a frying pan over medium–high heat. Add the coconut oil, garlic and asparagus, and season with salt and pepper. Cook for 2 minutes or until the asparagus is slightly tender.

Divide the asparagus between two serving plates, reserving the oil in the pan. Place the eggs on top of the asparagus. Sprinkle over the parmesan and reserved oil. Serve immediately.

BRUSSELS SPROUTS AND BACON HASH

Serves 4

8 slices lean bacon, trimmed and cut into small strips
300 g (10½ oz) button mushrooms, sliced
freshly ground black pepper
400 g (14 oz) brussels sprouts, thinly sliced
4 large eggs

Fry the bacon in a large non-stick frying pan over medium-high heat until cooked. Transfer to a plate and set aside.

Add the mushrooms to another non-stick frying pan. Cook over medium heat for 5-10 minutes or until they soften. Grind some black pepper over the mushrooms. When the mushrooms are browned, add the brussels sprouts and cook, stirring frequently, for 10-15 minutes or until the sprouts are tender. Stir in the bacon strips.

Create four indentations in the brussels sprout mixture and crack an egg into each one. Cook until the egg whites are set, then remove the pan from the heat and serve.

NOTES: Adding 1 teaspoon coconut oil when cooking the mushrooms will help tenderise them. If you prefer the egg yolks firm, cover the pan with a lid while the eggs are cooking, or transfer the pan to the oven to finish cooking.

CAULIFLOWER RISSOLES

Makes 8-10

250 g (9 oz/2 cups) cauliflower florets
1 egg, lightly beaten
¼ red onion, finely diced
2 tablespoons grated parmesan cheese
½ teaspoon onion powder
½ teaspoon garlic powder
½ teaspoon snipped chives
salt and freshly ground black pepper

Steam the cauliflower over a saucepan of boiling water until tender. Set aside to cool.

Mash the cooled cauliflower in a bowl. Add the remaining ingredients and mix until well combined. Using your hands, form the mixture into 8-10 patties.

Heat a non-stick frying pan over medium-high heat. Cook the patties for 3-5 minutes on each side or until golden brown. Serve warm or cold.

CARIBBEAN BEEF

Serves 6-8

1.5 kg (3 lb 5 oz) chuck steak, trimmed
1 onion, finely chopped
4 garlic cloves, crushed
1-2 fresh red chillies, finely chopped
2 bay leaves
1 rosemary sprig
1 tablespoon ground cumin
1 tablespoon dried oregano
¼ teaspoon ground cloves
salt and freshly ground black pepper
125 ml (4 fl oz/½ cup) low-sodium beef stock
3 tablespoons lime juice
2 tablespoons apple cider vinegar
2 shakes of Tabasco sauce

Heat a frying pan over medium-high heat and sear the beef all over. Transfer to a slow cooker.

Combine the remaining ingredients in a bowl. Pour over the meat in the slow cooker.

Turn on the slow cooker and leave to cook overnight (or while you're at work). Use two forks to shred the beef. Serve hot or portion up and store in the fridge for a week's worth of lunches, ready to go!

FOIL-ROASTED EGGPLANT

Serves 4

1 eggplant (aubergine), cut into chunks
stevia sweetener, to taste
ground cinnamon, to taste
salt and freshly ground black pepper
chilli flakes, to taste

Preheat the oven to 200°C (400°F).

Put the eggplant chunks on a sheet of foil. Sprinkle the eggplant with the stevia, cinnamon, salt, pepper and chilli flakes.

Wrap the eggplant in the foil to form a parcel and then bake for 30 minutes or until the eggplant is tender. Serve hot.

ZESTY LEMON GRILLED CALAMARI WITH GARLIC »

Serves 4

4 squid tubes, about 225 g (8 oz) each, cleaned
grated zest and juice of 1 lemon
2 garlic cloves, finely diced
1 tablespoon melted coconut oil
sea salt and freshly ground black pepper
coriander (cilantro) leaves, to garnish
lemon wedges, to serve

Rinse the squid and pat dry with paper towel. Cut each tube open by slicing down one side. Carefully score the inside of the flesh in a diamond pattern, without cutting all the way through.

Combine the lemon zest, lemon juice, garlic, coconut oil, salt and pepper in a bowl to make a marinade. Rub the marinade into the squid, cover with plastic wrap and marinate in the fridge for at least 2 hours.

Preheat a barbecue or non-stick frying pan over high heat. Cook the squid for about 2 minutes on each side or until the flesh curls and changes colour.

Serve the squid garnished with the coriander, and with lemon wedges for squeezing over the squid.

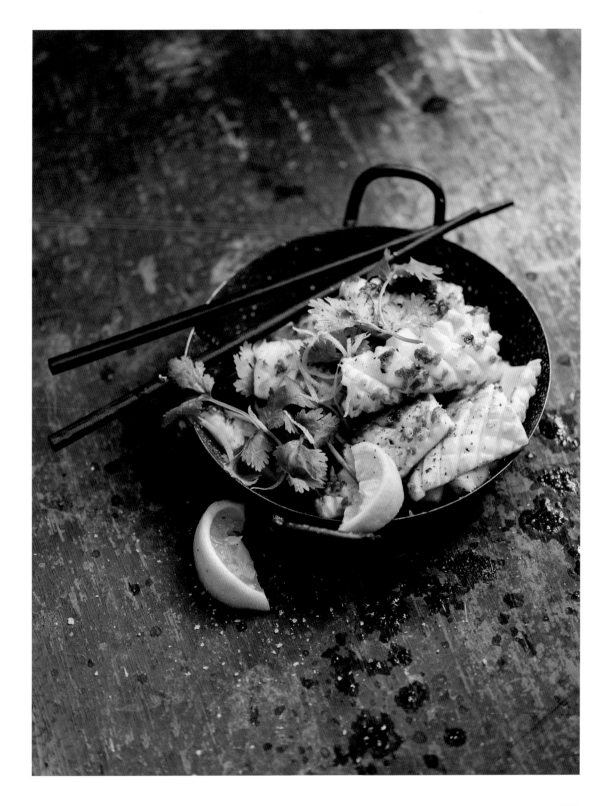

GRILLED SCALLOPS WRAPPED IN HAM

Makes 10

10 large scallops
freshly ground black pepper
5 slices ham off the bone or shaved ham

Rinse the scallops and pat dry with paper towel. Season with a little pepper.

Trim any fat off the ham slices and cut them in half. Wrap each scallop in a strip of ham and secure with a toothpick.

Preheat a barbecue grill to medium-high. Cook the scallops for 3 minutes on each side or until they are cooked through. Serve immediately.

EASY CHICKEN STIR-FRY »

Serves 4

500 g (1 lb 2 oz) skinless chicken thigh fillets, cut into strips
1 red onion, sliced
2 garlic cloves, crushed
1 tablespoon finely chopped fresh ginger
1 small fresh red chilli, seeded and chopped
1 red capsicum (pepper), sliced
1 green capsicum (pepper), sliced
115 g (4 oz/1 cup) bean sprouts, trimmed
2 tablespoons salt-reduced soy sauce
2 tablespoons lime juice
salt and freshly ground black pepper

Heat a large non-stick frying pan or wok over medium-high heat. Stir-fry the chicken until browned all over and cooked through. Transfer to a bowl.

Add the onion, garlic, ginger and chilli to the pan and stir-fry for 2-3 minutes or until fragrant.

Add the capsicum and stir-fry for 2 minutes, then add the bean sprouts, soy sauce and chicken. Cook until the vegetables are tender but still crisp.

Sprinkle with the lime juice, then remove from the heat and season with salt and pepper. Serve hot.

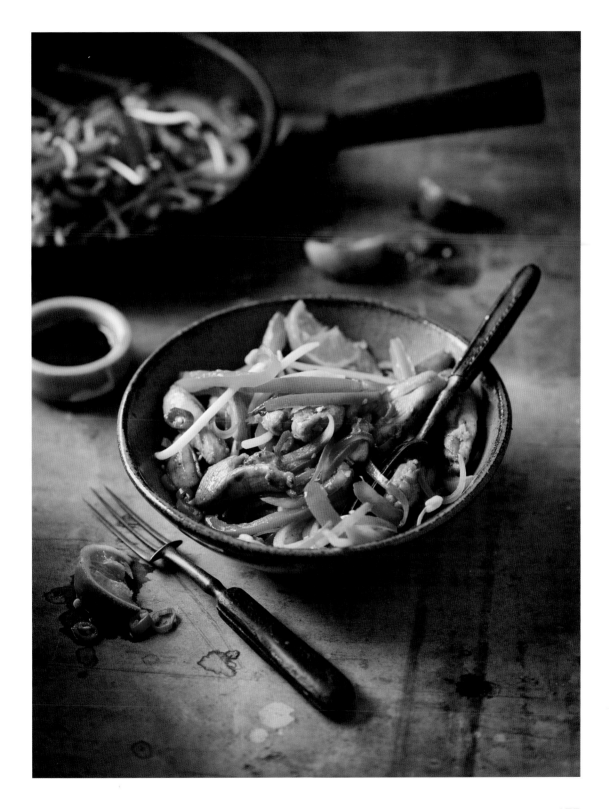

CHICKEN CURRY IN A HURRY

Serves 4

4 skinless chicken breast fillets, cut into
    bite-sized pieces
low-fat, low-carb plain yoghurt, to serve

Curry sauce
1 red capsicum (pepper), cut into chunks
2–3 spring onions (scallions), cut into short lengths,
    a little reserved and finely sliced, for garnish
1 bunch coriander (cilantro), a few leaves reserved
    for garnish
2 garlic cloves
3 cm (1¼ inch) piece fresh ginger
1 small fresh red chilli
2 tablespoons curry powder
1 tablespoon ground turmeric
1 tablespoon stevia
1 tablespoon low-sodium chicken stock or water

To make the curry sauce, put all the ingredients in a high-powered blender. Add 1–2 tablespoons water and blend to a paste, adding more water if needed.

Heat a large non-stick frying pan over medium heat. Stir-fry the chicken pieces for 5–8 minutes or until browned and almost cooked. Stir in the curry sauce and simmer for 10 minutes or until the chicken is cooked through, adding a little water if it starts to stick.

Serve the curry with a dollop of yoghurt, sprinkled with the reserved coriander leaves and spring onion.

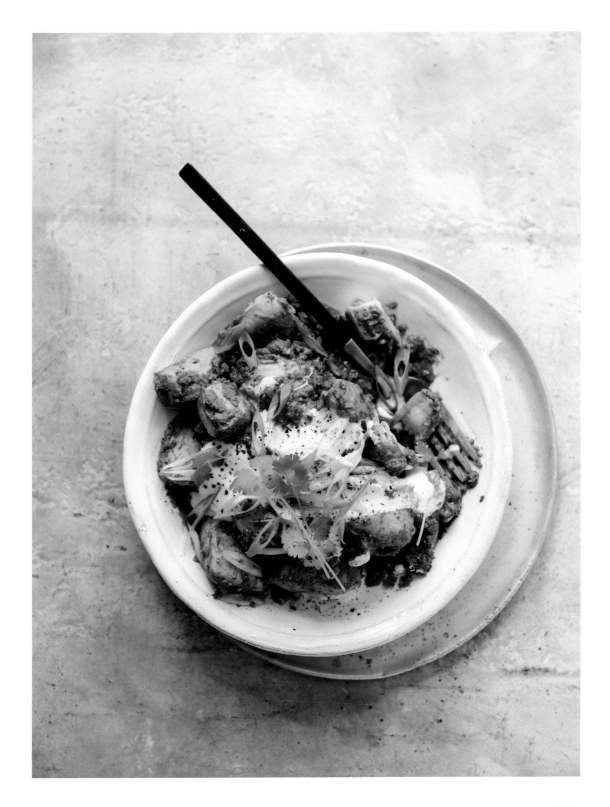

WEEK 5
RECIPES

SMASHED AVOCADO AND FETA ON PROTEIN BREAD

Serves 4

1 ripe avocado
juice of 1 lime
1–2 teaspoons chopped coriander (cilantro) leaves
1 fresh green chilli, chopped
salt and freshly ground black pepper
60 g (2¼ oz) low-fat feta cheese, crumbled
4 slices Protein bread (from The Protein Bread Co.), toasted

Cut the avocado in half and remove the stone. Scoop the flesh into a bowl and add the lime juice, coriander and chilli. Season well with salt and pepper, then mash the mixture together with a fork, leaving some larger chunks. Taste and add more seasoning if needed.

Stir in half the feta, then spoon the mixture onto the toasted protein bread. Scatter the remaining feta over the top and serve.

ZUCCHINI AND RICOTTA FRITTATA

Serves 4

2 zucchini (courgettes)
1 tablespoon salt, plus extra to season
4 eggs
2 garlic cloves, crushed
1-2 tablespoons chopped mint leaves (optional)
125 g (4½ oz) low-fat ricotta cheese, crumbled
freshly ground black pepper
8 cherry tomatoes
basil leaves, to serve

Preheat the grill (broiler) to medium-high.

Coarsely grate the zucchini and squeeze out as much liquid as possible. Transfer to a bowl and stir in the salt.

Lightly whisk the eggs, garlic and mint (if using) in a large bowl. Gently fold in the zucchini, then fold in the crumbled ricotta. Season with salt and freshly ground pepper.

Heat a non-stick ovenproof frying pan over medium heat. Pour in the zucchini mixture and cook for about 5-6 minutes or until the edge is set, but the centre is runny. Put the pan under the preheated grill, about 6 cm (2½ inches) away from the heat. Cook the frittata for 3 minutes or until it is just set and the top is golden brown.

Serve a couple of slices of frittata with the cherry tomatoes and basil leaves.

DEVIL NACHOS

Serves 4

500 g (1 lb 2 oz) extra-lean minced (ground) beef
1 onion, diced
2 teaspoons crushed garlic
30 g (1 oz) Mexican seasoning
ground cumin, to taste
smoked paprika, to taste
2 tomatoes, diced
salt and freshly ground black pepper

Nacho chips
330 g (11¹/₂ oz) packet Protein bread mix
    (from The Protein Bread Co.)
2 extra large eggs or 100 ml (3¹/₂ fl oz) egg whites
1 tablespoon white vinegar
smoked paprika, for sprinkling

To serve
chopped fresh red chilli (optional)
diced avocado
lime wedges

Line a baking tray with baking paper. Preheat the oven to 220°C (425°F).

To make the nacho chips, prepare the bread mix according to the packet instructions with the eggs or egg whites, vinegar and 440 ml (15¹/₄ fl oz/1³/₄ cups) water. Thinly spread a layer of the mixture on the prepared tray and sprinkle with smoked paprika. Bake for 10 minutes. Remove the tray from the oven and slice the nacho chips into small triangles. Spread them out on the tray and bake until golden brown and crunchy.

Heat a frying pan over medium–high heat. Add the beef, onion, garlic, Mexican seasoning, cumin and paprika. Cook, stirring and breaking up any lumps, for 5 minutes or until the beef is cooked. Add the diced tomato and 250 ml (9 fl oz/1 cup) water. Season well, then reduce the heat and simmer until the mixture has thickened.

Arrange the nacho chips on a plate and top with the beef mixture, chilli (if using), avocado and lime wedges. Serve immediately.

CHICKEN AND VEGETABLE CASSEROLE

Serves 1 (see Note)

150 ml (5½ fl oz) skim or non-fat milk

2 tablespoons Philadelphia light cream for cooking

1 tablespoon grated parmesan cheese, plus extra
   for sprinkling

1 teaspoon Italian seasoning

salt and freshly ground black pepper

120 g (4¼ oz/2 cups) broccoli florets

1 zucchini (courgette), chopped

150 g (5½ oz/2 cups) shredded cabbage

350 g (12 oz) skinless chicken thigh or breast fillet, diced

2 red capsicums (peppers), chopped

basil leaves, to serve (optional)

NOTE: IT'S WELL WORTH SCALING THIS RECIPE UP TO MAKE LUNCHES OR DINNERS FOR THE WEEK AHEAD.

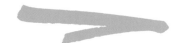

Preheat the oven to 200°C (400°F).

Combine the milk and cream in a saucepan over low heat. Cook, stirring, until slightly thickened. Add the parmesan and Italian seasoning, and season with salt and pepper. Cook, stirring, until thickened, watching to make sure it doesn't burn. Remove from the heat and set aside.

Cook the broccoli, zucchini and cabbage in a steamer over a saucepan of boiling water until bright green and just tender.

Meanwhile, cook the diced chicken in a non-stick frying pan over medium-high heat for 5 minutes or until browned. Transfer to an ovenproof dish and combine with the steamed vegetables and capsicum.

Pour the sauce over the chicken and vegetables and sprinkle grated parmesan over the top. Bake for 20-30 minutes or until lightly browned. Serve hot, sprinkled with basil leaves (if using).

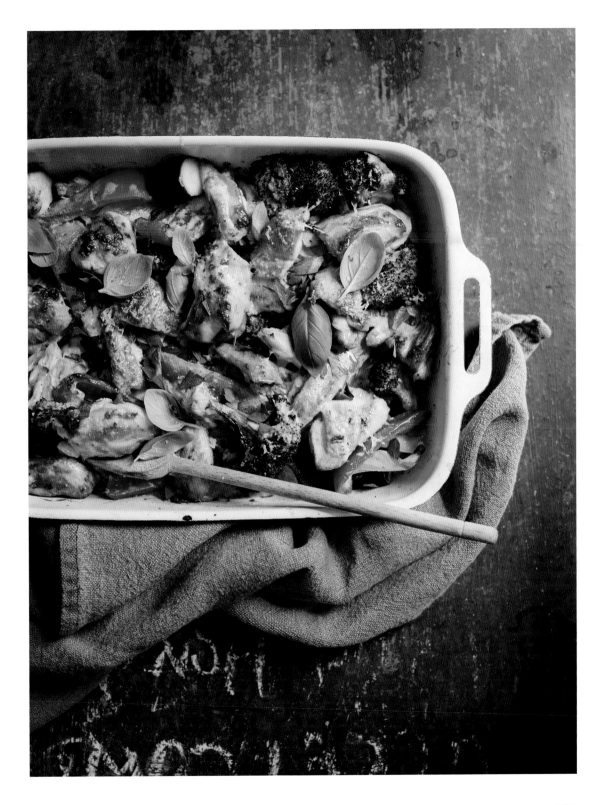

COTTAGE CHEESE DEVILLED EGGS

Makes 4

2 hard-boiled eggs, cooled
2 tablespoons low-fat cottage cheese
2 teaspoons dijon or other mustard
salt and freshly ground black pepper
paprika, for sprinkling

Peel the eggs and halve them lengthways, then scoop out the yolks and put them in a bowl. Set the egg whites aside.

Add the cottage cheese and mustard to the egg yolks, and mash them together. Season with salt and freshly ground black pepper.

Spoon the egg yolk mixture into the egg white halves and sprinkle with paprika to serve.

PULLED PORK SALAD »

Serves 1–2

250 g (9 oz) packet ready-made pulled pork
5 cherry tomatoes, halved
½ Lebanese (short) cucumber, peeled into ribbons
1–2 tablespoons crumbled low-fat feta cheese
60 g (2¼ oz) mixed baby English spinach and
    rocket (arugula)
micro herbs, to garnish (optional)

Heat the pork following the packet instructions.

Toss the hot pork with the tomato, cucumber, feta, spinach and rocket. Serve immediately, garnished with micro herbs (if using).

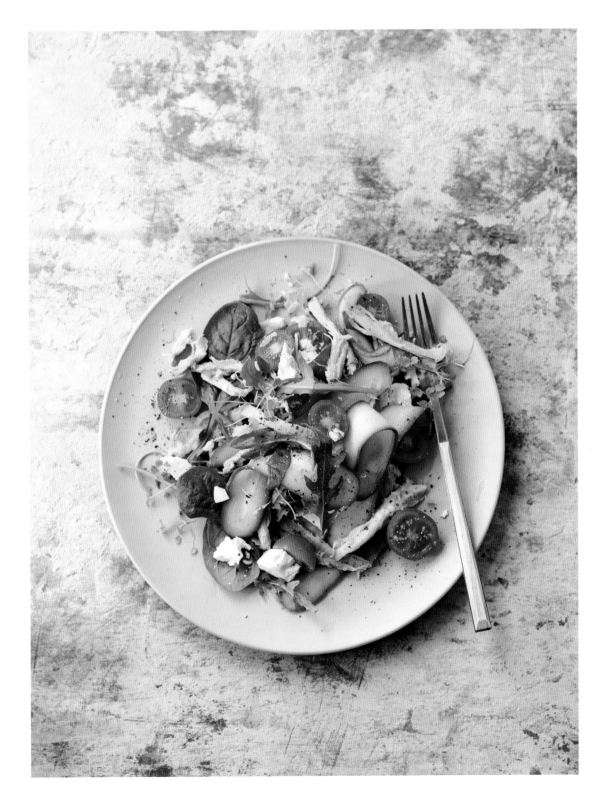

WEEK 6
RECIPES

HUEVOS A LA RANCHERA

Serves 4

½ onion, diced
1 garlic clove, crushed
2 ripe tomatoes, chopped
½ green capsicum (pepper), chopped
salt-reduced soy sauce, to taste
salt and freshly ground black pepper
juice of ½ lime
chilli flakes, to taste
4 eggs
coriander (cilantro) leaves, to serve

Heat a non-stick frying pan over medium heat. Cook the onion and garlic until the onion is translucent and aromatic.

Add the tomato and capsicum, then stir in the soy sauce, salt, pepper, lime juice and chilli flakes, to taste. Bring to a simmer and cook for about 3 minutes or until the tomato has softened.

Meanwhile, fry the eggs in another non-stick frying pan until done to your liking.

Transfer the eggs to a plate, then pour the tomato mixture over the top and sprinkle with the coriander to serve.

BACON AND EGG CUPS

Makes 6

6 slices shoulder bacon
6 eggs
30 g (1 oz) low-fat feta cheese, crumbled

Preheat the oven to 180°C (350°F).

Line six holes of a silicone muffin tray with the bacon slices. Crack one egg into each muffin hole and then sprinkle with the feta.

Bake for 25–30 minutes or until the bacon is cooked and the eggs are done to your liking.

NOTE: THESE ARE GREAT REHEATED OR SERVED COLD, SO MAKE EXTRA FOR EASY BREAKFASTS OR SNACKS.

2015 Hella yeah salad

Serves 1

100 g (3½ oz) chopped lettuce
50 g (1¾ oz) red capsicum (pepper), diced or thinly sliced
4 button or small mushrooms, thinly sliced
50 g (1¾ oz) low-fat feta cheese, crumbled
6 anchovy fillets

Roasted garlic dressing
6 roasted garlic cloves
2 tablespoons extra-light cream cheese
2 tablespoons apple cider vinegar

Combine the lettuce, capsicum, mushrooms, feta and anchovies in a bowl.

To make the dressing, squeeze the roasted garlic flesh into a small screw-top jar and discard the skin. Add the cream cheese and vinegar to the jar and shake until well combined.

Drizzle the dressing over the salad and serve.

NOTE: YOU CAN REPLACE THE FETA WITH GRATED PARMESAN CHEESE. ADD SOME DICED, COOKED CHICKEN TO MAKE HELLA CHOOK YEAH SALAD.

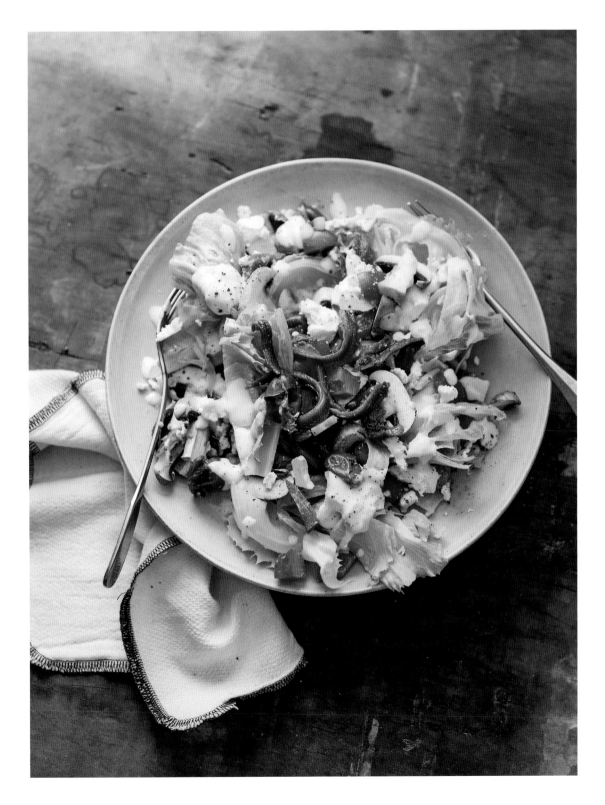

SAUTÉED SPINACH

Serves 4

2 tablespoons chopped garlic
700 g (1 lb 9 oz) baby English spinach
2 teaspoons salt
freshly ground black pepper
low-fat feta or cottage cheese, to serve
lemon wedges, to serve

Sauté the garlic in a frying pan over medium-low heat until aromatic but not browned. Add the spinach, salt and a good grinding of black pepper and cook, stirring, until the spinach is coated with the garlic. Cover and cook for 2–3 minutes or until the spinach is starting to wilt.

Increase the heat and cook, uncovered, for 2 minutes or until the spinach has wilted and halved in volume.

Using a slotted spoon, transfer the sautéd spinach to a plate. Sprinkle with the feta or cottage cheese and some salt, if needed, and serve hot with the lemon wedges.

THYME SALMON FILLETS

Serves 2

2 salmon fillets
salt and freshly ground black pepper
8 thyme sprigs

Preheat the oven to 250°C (500°F). Line a baking tray with baking paper.

Rinse the salmon fillets and pat dry. Rub all over with salt and pepper. Place the thyme sprigs on the baking tray and place the salmon on top.

Turn off the oven and immediately place the salmon inside. Leave for 10–12 minutes or until the salmon is just pink on the very inside.

Serve the hot salmon with salad or vegetables.

FISHY RISSOLES

Makes 12

750 g (1 lb 10 oz) redfish fillets, roughly chopped
1 tablespoon Thai red curry paste
coriander (cilantro) leaves, to taste

Put the fish, curry paste and coriander leaves in a food processor. Blend until the mixture forms a paste. Shape the fish mixture into 12 rissoles.

Heat a large non-stick frying pan over medium–high heat. Cook the rissoles in batches for 3–4 minutes on each side or until cooked through, turning once. Serve hot or cold.

SUPER-EASY PERI-PERI CHICKEN

Serves 1

1 small skinless chicken breast fillet
peri-peri spice mix
all-purpose seasoning
2 handfuls baby English spinach
1 Lebanese (short) cucumber, thinly sliced
low-carb plain yoghurt, to serve

Preheat the oven to 180°C (350°F). Line a small baking tray with baking paper.

Sprinkle the chicken with the spices, to taste. Place the chicken on the tray and bake for 20 minutes or until cooked through.

Slice the chicken and serve on a bed of baby spinach and cucumber. Serve drizzled with the yoghurt (it will help cool down the chicken if you added too much peri-peri spice).

THAI GREEN CURRY CHICKEN BALLS

Serves 2

300 g (10½ oz) skinless chicken thigh fillets
80 g (2¾ oz) English spinach
½ onion, diced
2 garlic cloves, diced
1 long fresh green chilli, chopped
2 teaspoons grated fresh ginger
20 g (¾ oz) coriander (cilantro) leaves and stems
1 egg white
¼ teaspoon ground black pepper
1 teaspoon chilli flakes
½ teaspoon ground coriander
½ teaspoon ground cumin
sprinkle of ground turmeric
sprinkle of ground paprika
lime wedges, for serving

Chop the chicken in a food processor. Add the remaining ingredients and pulse until the mixture forms a paste.

Heat a non-stick frying pan over medium–high heat. Drop heaped teaspoons of the chicken mixture into the pan and fry in batches for about 5 minutes or until cooked through and golden brown. Serve hot or cold with lime wedges for squeezing over.

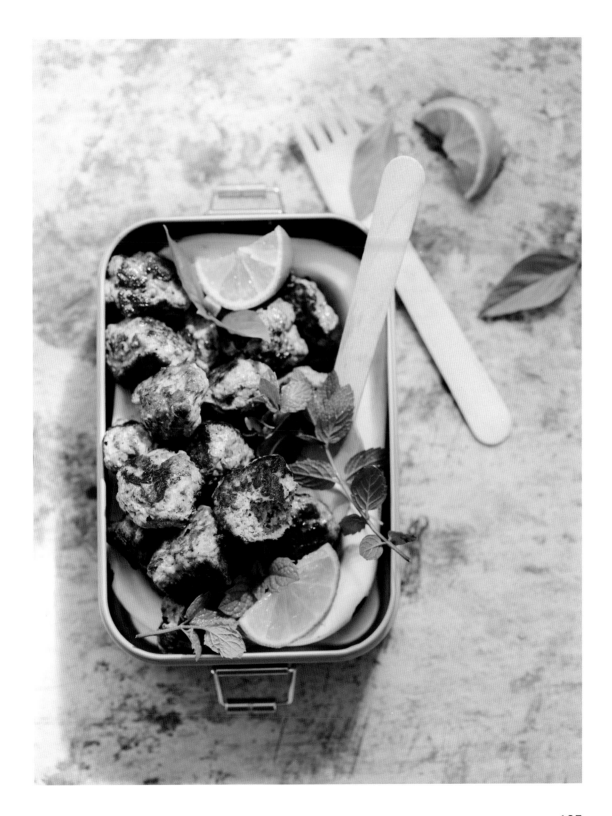

WEEK 7
RECIPES

PORK AND FENNEL PATTIES

Makes 4

2 teaspoons fennel seeds
1 small onion, finely diced
500 g (1 lb 2 oz) extra-lean minced (ground) pork
3 tablespoons extra-light mozzarella cheese
1 egg, lightly beaten
1 teaspoon mustard powder
2 tablespoons chia seeds (optional)
2 teaspoons dried garlic granules

Dipping sauce
1/2 teaspoon dried chives
3 tablespoons extra-light sour cream

Dry-fry the fennel seeds in a non-stick frying pan over medium-high heat until fragrant. Add the onion and cook, stirring, until the onion is softened and browned. Transfer to a bowl and wipe out the frying pan.

Add the pork, mozzarella, egg, mustard powder and chia seeds (if using) to the onion and mix until well combined. Shape the mixture into 4 patties.

Cook the patties in the frying pan over medium-high heat for 5 minutes. Sprinkle with the garlic granules, pressing them into the patties, then turn and cook for another 5 minutes or until cooked through.

To make the dipping sauce, stir the chives through the sour cream until well combined.

Serve the hot patties with the dipping sauce.

BUTTERFLY CHICKEN WITH ROSEMARY

Serves 1

1 skinless chicken breast fillet
2 teaspoons sea salt flakes or rock salt
large pinch of freshly ground black pepper
2 teaspoons finely chopped rosemary
1 teaspoon lemon juice

Butterfly the chicken breast by cutting it in half horizontally, without cutting all the way through, then open out.

Dissolve the salt flakes or rock salt in 250 ml (9 fl oz/1 cup) water in a bowl. Add the chicken and set aside for 5–10 minutes, then remove from the salt water. Rub vigorously with the pepper and rosemary.

Heat a non-stick frying pan over high heat until it begins to smoke. Pan-fry the chicken for 4–5 minutes, turning every 30 seconds until it is cooked through. Sprinkle the lemon juice over the chicken and serve immediately.

ASPARAGUS, BACON AND RICOTTA FRITTATAS »

Makes 12

6 eggs
100 ml (3½ fl oz) skim or non-fat milk
smoked paprika, to taste (optional)
6 asparagus spears, chopped
6 rashers lean shortcut bacon, trimmed and chopped
3 tablespoons low-fat ricotta cheese

Preheat the oven to 160°C (320°F). Lightly grease a 12-hole muffin tin.

Whisk the eggs, milk and paprika (if using). Set aside.

Heat a frying pan over medium-high heat. Cook the asparagus for 2–3 minutes or until slightly soft. Remove from the pan and set aside.

Add the bacon to the pan and fry until cooked through.

Add equal amounts of the bacon and asparagus to each muffin hole. Pour the egg mixture into the holes and finish with a small spoonful of ricotta.

Bake the frittatas for 20 minutes or until set. Serve hot or cold.

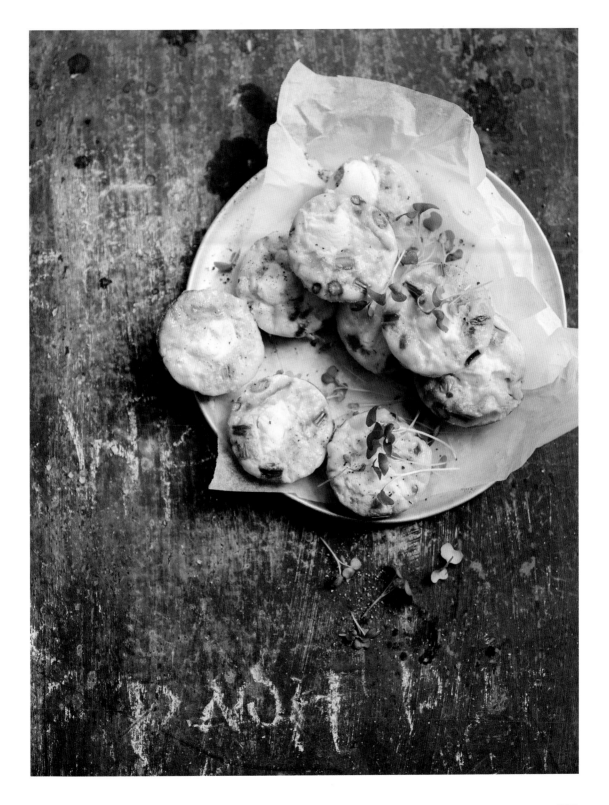

SWEET ONION MEATBALLS

Makes 8-12

1 small onion, diced
1 teaspoon Tuscan, herbes de Provençe, Mexican or
    Indian spice blend
salt and freshly ground black pepper
400 g lean minced (ground) beef, chicken, lamb or pork
2 egg yolks
canola oil spray

Heat a frying pan over medium heat and add 1 teaspoon water. Cook the onion, stirring, until translucent. Add the spice blend and season with salt and pepper. Transfer to a bowl and wipe out the frying pan.

Add the meat and egg yolks to the onion. Using wet hands, mix until combined, then shape the mixture into 8-12 meatballs.

Spray the frying pan with canola oil, then add the meatballs and cook for about 10 minutes, turning them every few minutes until they are golden brown and cooked through. Serve hot or cold.

NOTE: YOU CAN USE A COMBINATION OF DIFFERENT MEATS IN THESE MEATBALLS. ORGANIC MEAT IS MUCH JUICIER AND TASTES BETTER. THE MEATBALLS ARE GREAT SERVED HOT ON A BED OF BABY ENGLISH SPINACH OR SERVED COLD AS A LUNCHBOX SNACK.

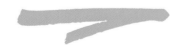

SAUSAGE ROLLS

Makes 6–8

Pastry

½ packet (115 g/4 oz) Protein bread mix
    (from The Protein Bread Co.)
2 egg whites

Filling

250 g (9 oz) extra-lean minced (ground) pork
½ onion, diced
1 tablespoon finely diced garlic
1 tablespoon finely diced fresh ginger
1 tablespoon salt-reduced soy sauce
pinch of salt
pinch of freshly ground black pepper

Preheat the oven to 180°C (350°F). Line a large baking tray with baking paper.

To make the pastry, prepare the bread mix with the egg whites and 225 ml (7½ fl oz) water according to the packet instructions, but only leave the mixture to thicken for about 5 minutes. Press the mixture onto the baking tray as flat and thin as you can. Bake for about 10 minutes or until the pastry is starting to firm up.

Meanwhile, mix all of the filling ingredients together in a bowl until well combined.

Arrange the filling in a line along the middle of the pastry, then wrap the pastry around the filling. Bake for about 10 minutes, then remove from the oven and slice into 6–8 pieces. Return the sausage rolls to the oven for a further 10–15 minutes or until just cooked through. Serve hot or cold.

NOTE: Do not overcook the sausage rolls or the pork will dry out. For an extra golden finish, brush a little egg over the pastry before baking the sausage rolls.

BARBECUED CHICKEN TIKKA KEBABS

Serves 2

2 skinless chicken breast fillets
100 g (3½ oz) low-carb fat-free plain yoghurt
1 tablespoon lemon juice
2 teaspoons minced ginger
1 teaspoon minced garlic
2 teaspoons ground coriander
cayenne pepper, to taste

Cut the chicken into 3 cm (1¼ inch) cubes.

Combine the yoghurt, lemon juice, ginger, garlic, coriander and cayenne pepper in a glass or plastic container with a lid. Add the chicken cubes to the marinade and toss to coat. Cover and refrigerate overnight.

Preheat a barbecue or grill (broiler) to high.

Thread the marinated chicken cubes onto bamboo or metal skewers. Cook the kebabs on the hot barbecue or under the grill, turning frequently, for 8–10 minutes or until the chicken is cooked through. Serve on a bed of salad.

NOTE: IF YOU'RE USING BAMBOO SKEWERS, SOAK THEM IN WATER FOR 30 MINUTES BEFORE THREADING THE CHICKEN. THIS WILL HELP PREVENT THEM FROM BURNING.

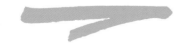

GRILLED CURRIED FISH

Serves 2

2 fish fillets, skin on
salt and freshly ground black pepper
2 spring onions (scallions), thinly sliced
3 tablespoons curry powder
1 teaspoon chilli powder or chilli flakes
2 teaspoons salt-reduced soy sauce
juice of ½ lime

Season the fish with salt and pepper.

Combine the spring onion, curry powder, chilli, soy sauce and lime juice in a bowl and mix to a thick paste. Spread the paste on the skinless side of the fish.

Heat a non-stick frying pan over medium heat. Add the fish, skin side down, and cook for 4 minutes. Turn and cook for another 4 minutes or until the fish starts to flake. Serve hot.

NOTE: USE COD OR OTHER FIRM FISH FILLETS. YOU CAN ALSO BARBECUE OR GRILL (BROIL) THE FISH. SERVE THE FISH WITH LOW-CARB, LOW-FAT GREEK-STYLE YOGHURT OR PLAIN YOGHURT, OR EXTRA-LIGHT SOUR CREAM.

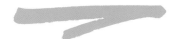

BEEF SCHNITZEL WITH MUSHROOM SAUCE

Serves 4

4 beef fillets
1 egg, lightly beaten
4 French shallots, finely diced
2–3 mushrooms, thinly sliced
2–3 thyme sprigs, leaves only
1 tablespoon extra-light cream cheese
freshly ground black pepper

Preheat the oven to 180°C (350°F). Line a baking tray with baking paper.

Using a meat tenderiser, flatten the beef fillets to form 1 cm (½ inch) thick schnitzels.

Dip the schnitzels in the beaten egg. Place on the baking tray and bake for about 15 minutes or until golden.

Meanwhile, put the diced shallots and 3 tablespoons water in a saucepan and sauté over medium-high heat for 5 minutes or until the shallots are soft. Add the mushrooms, thyme and another 3 tablespoons water. Cook over medium heat for 5–10 minutes or until the mushrooms are cooked through.

Remove the pan from the heat. Add the cream cheese and pepper, to taste. Stir until the sauce is blended and smooth. Return to the heat and simmer over medium heat until the sauce has reduced to your desired thickness.

Spoon the mushroom sauce over the hot schnitzels.

NOTE: YOU CAN FRY THE SCHNITZELS IN A FRYING PAN FOR 2-3 MINUTES ON EACH SIDE INSTEAD OF BAKING THEM. THE PEPPER CAN BE SUBSTITUTED WITH PAPRIKA.

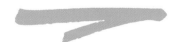

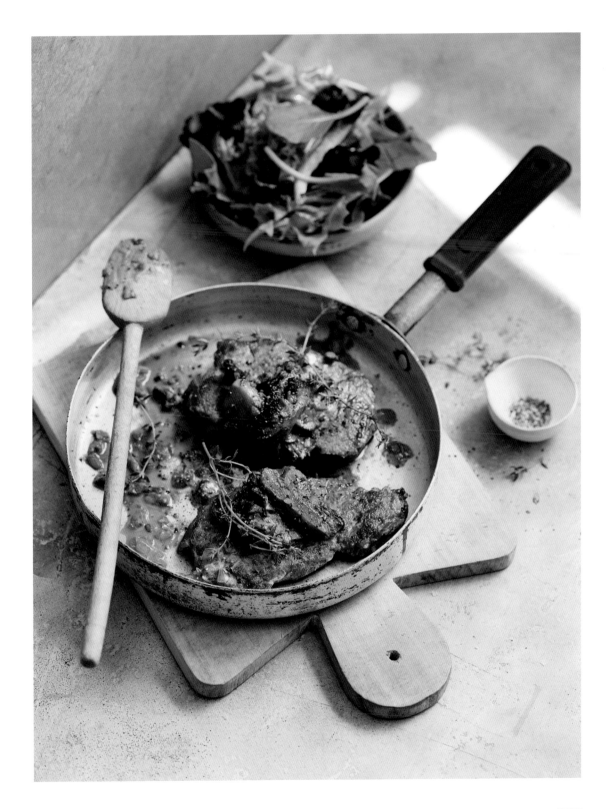

WEEK 8
RECIPES

MINT CURRY OMELETTE

Serves 2

4 eggs
50 g (1¾ oz) extra-light ricotta or cream cheese
1–2 teaspoons curry powder
1–2 tablespoons mint leaves
salt and freshly ground black pepper

Beat the eggs with the ricotta or cream cheese in a bowl until combined. Fold in the curry powder and mint, and season with salt and pepper.

Heat a non-stick frying pan over low heat. Pour in the egg mixture and cook until the omelette is set, then turn and cook the other side until golden. Serve hot.

CAULIFLOWER FRIED RICE

Serves 6

1 cauliflower, cut into florets
¼ cabbage, diced
3 carrots, diced
½ zucchini (courgette), diced
¼ red capsicum (pepper), diced
¼ green capsicum (pepper), diced
¼ yellow capsicum (pepper), diced
100 g (3½ oz) mushrooms, diced
4–6 asparagus spears, cut into 2.5 cm (1 inch) pieces
4 slices lean shortcut bacon, trimmed and cut into strips
2 eggs
pinch of Chinese five spice
salt and freshly ground black pepper
salt-reduced soy sauce, to taste
chives, for serving

NOTE: FOR A MORE SUBSTANTIAL MEAL, ADD SOME COOKED CHICKEN, PRAWNS (SHRIMP) OR OTHER PROTEIN OF YOUR CHOICE.

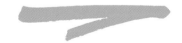

Put the cauliflower florets in a food processor and pulse until they resemble rice grains.

Heat a large non-stick frying pan over medium-high heat. Add the cabbage, carrot, zucchini, capsicum, mushroom, asparagus and cauliflower and sauté until tender. Remove the vegetables from the pan and set aside.

Cook the bacon in the same pan over medium-high heat until golden. Remove from the pan and set aside.

Whisk the eggs in a bowl, then pour into the hot pan and cook over medium-high heat for 2–3 minutes or until set and golden, then turn and cook the other side for a further 2–3 minutes or until set and golden. Remove from the pan and cut into 2.5 cm (1 inch) strips.

Wipe out the pan or use a large wok. Add the vegetables, bacon and egg and cook, tossing, until warmed through. Add the Chinese five spice, salt, pepper and a dash of soy sauce. Serve warm with some finely chopped chives sprinkled on top.

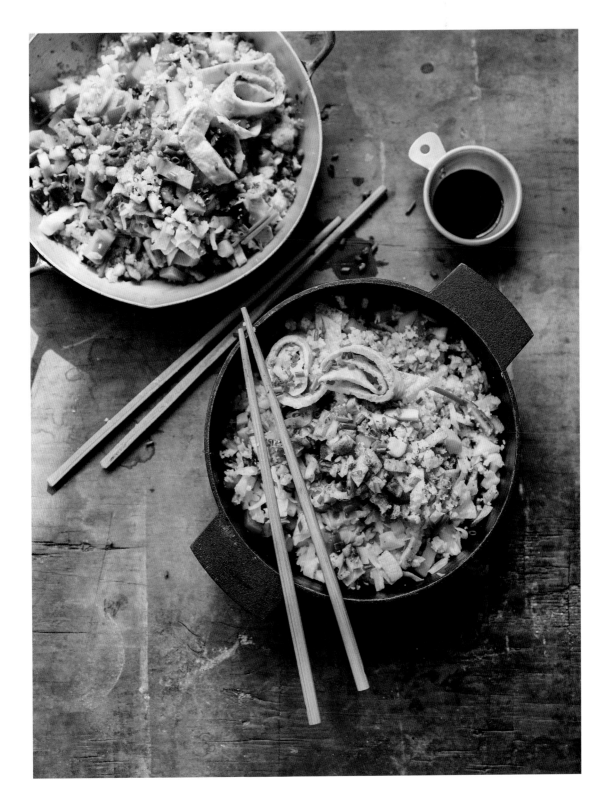

TACO-LESS TACOS
Serves 4

4 large flat mushrooms
salt
1 small onion, diced
500 g (1 lb 2 oz) lean minced (ground) beef, pork or chicken
1 teaspoon crushed garlic
1 teaspoon paprika
1 teaspoon ground cumin
1 teaspoon dried oregano
1 teaspoon chilli powder
1 teaspoon ground coriander
300 g (10½ oz) jar tomato salsa

To serve
1 Lebanese (short) cucumber, diced
1 carrot, grated
½ red capsicum (pepper), diced
1 avocado, diced
shredded lettuce
grated low-fat cheddar cheese
low-fat sour cream

Preheat the oven to 180°C (350°F). Place the mushrooms on a wire rack on a baking tray, sprinkle with salt and bake for 15 minutes, then turn and sprinkle with more salt. Bake for a further 15 minutes or until the mushrooms are cooked and slightly dried out.

Meanwhile, heat a large non-stick frying pan over medium heat. Cook the onion until translucent, then add the meat and cook, stirring and breaking up any lumps, for 5 minutes or until browned. Carefully drain the fat from the pan.

Stir in the spices and half the salsa, then simmer over low heat while the mushrooms finish cooking. Add more salsa or water if the mixture is drying out.

Turn the mushrooms upside down on serving plates and serve topped with the meat, toppings and remaining salsa.

NOTE: YOU CAN USE MEXICAN SEASONING INSTEAD OF THE SPICES TO FLAVOUR THE MEAT.

POMMY SCOTCH EGGS

Makes 5

6 eggs
500 g (1 lb 2 oz) lean minced (ground) turkey
salt and freshly ground black pepper

Add five of the eggs to a saucepan of water and cook over medium-high heat for 7-8 minutes or until they are almost hard-boiled. Drain and cool, then remove the shells.

Preheat the oven to 180°C (350°F). Line a baking tray with baking paper.

Lightly beat the remaining egg, then mix with the turkey. Season with salt and pepper.

Divide the turkey mixture into five portions. Mould each portion around an egg.

Put the Scotch eggs on the tray and bake for 15 minutes. Drain any excess fat, turn the eggs and cook for another 15 minutes. Drain the eggs on paper towel before serving hot or cold.

BACON AND AVOCADO FRIES

Serves 4

1 avocado
6 slices lean bacon

Preheat the oven to 200°C (400°F). Line a baking tray with baking paper and place a wire rack on top.

Cut the avocado into 12 thin strips. Cut each bacon slice in half to make 12 strips (leave a little of the fat on the bacon to flavour the avocado as it will melt away during cooking). Tightly wrap each avocado strip with a bacon strip and place on the wire rack.

Bake the fries until the bacon turns golden. Allow to cool slightly before serving.

GRILLED BEEF, SWEET POTATO AND ROCKET SALAD

Serves 4

500 g (1 lb 2 oz) sirloin steak
olive oil spray
300 g (10½ oz) orange sweet potato, thinly sliced
4 zucchini (courgettes), thinly sliced
¼ red onion, sliced
salt and freshly ground black pepper
grated zest and juice of 1 lemon
olive oil, to serve
160 g (5½ oz) rocket (arugula)
parmesan cheese, to serve
balsamic or apple cider vinegar, to serve

Preheat a barbecue grill to high or heat a chargrill pan over high heat. Cook the steak until done to your liking. Remove from the heat and loosely cover with foil to rest.

Lightly spray the sweet potato, zucchini and onion with olive oil. Cook on the barbecue or in the chargrill pan until lightly browned and tender. Season with salt and pepper.

Combine the lemon zest and juice with a little salt and pepper in a bowl. Add the vegetables and toss to coat. Sprinkle with olive oil.

Thinly slice the beef and add it to the vegetables. Gently toss to combine.

Serve the salad on a bed of rocket, topped with a shaving of parmesan and a drizzle of vinegar.

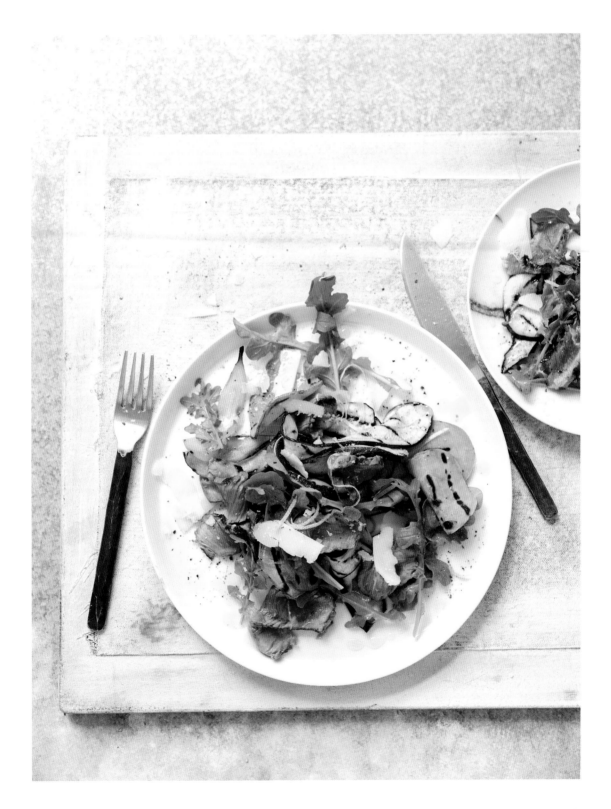

YOU MADE IT!

Congratulations on completing your 8 Weeks to Wow transformation! I am always astounded by what can be achieved when you really put your mind to something. Over the years I have been lucky enough to see thousands of successful transformations on the 8WTW program, and I always feel like a proud mother hen when another participant achieves his or her goal through hard work and persistence.

However, what I always like to remind people of is this: you can do so much more! Consider the last 8 weeks as a warm-up – the preparation, the pre-game show. And the best parts are yet to be revealed. You can go so much further than you've already gone. Every step you take is a step towards a bigger one. All the small steps add up to a great distance, as long as you keep moving forward.

Hopefully in the last 8 weeks you have learned a lot about what you need to eat and drink in order to perform, look and feel the best you possibly can. It's for a happier and healthier you. This journey has been about learning how to eat healthy, unprocessed foods, controlling your portion sizes and even the way that you perceive food. You don't need to completely remove the treat foods from your life, although it's likely that your tastebuds have changed a little throughout the challenge. Do you wonder why you don't crave the things you used to? Or, if you do still crave them, how much smaller or controlled the amount that you consume is?

This transformation is about not feeling guilty about having a high-sugar or high-fat treat if you feel that you want one. The basis of the program is about cutting everything back to the bare basics and working things back in so that you can be the best and healthiest version of yourself. You train your body to like good foods in exactly the same way as you train it to like bad foods, so remember to make good choices.

If you're beating yourself up about not achieving what you wanted to, going off track or not being able to train due to illness or injury, stop! We all beat ourselves up sometimes, it's just human nature. But try not to do it. I once read that self-criticism, although sometimes good for you, is akin to walking around with a mean person inside your head, who constantly grinds you down and criticises you until you actually start to believe you are no good. Ultimately, if you hear these negative things enough, that's where you'll end up.

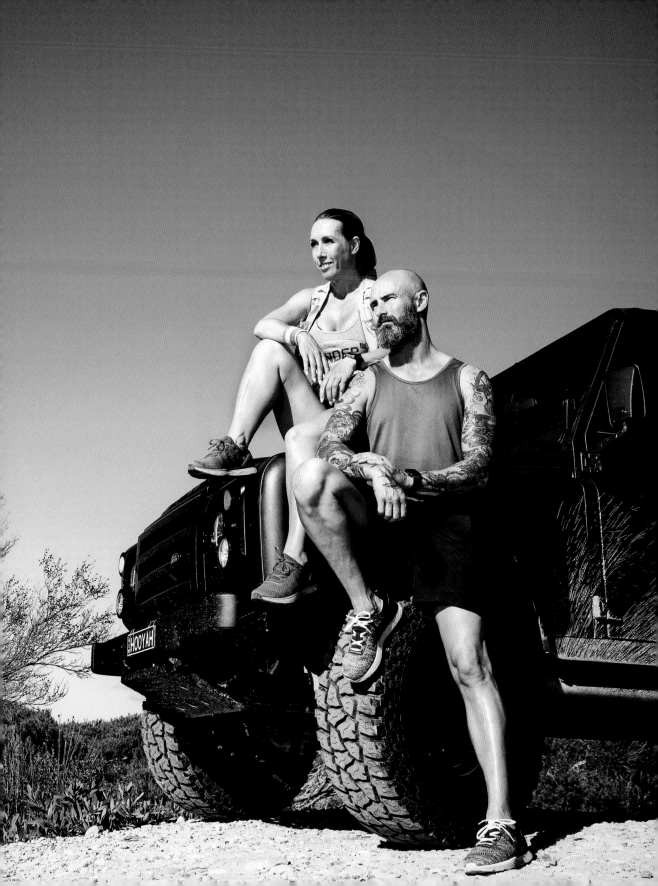

What I recommend is this: stop questioning if you could have done better and tell any doubts to go away, then start thinking about one thing that you did today that you could congratulate yourself on – something you did right. Maybe you ate something healthy instead of a chocolate bar, maybe you didn't go back for a second serving or got through a really tough training session. Maybe it was as simple as drinking your allocated water for the day.

The best thing about this book is that you can close it, turn it back to the first page, and do it over again, at your leisure. Your pace will differ from that of other people, so remember to be kind to yourself and try to implement one healthier aspect into your life at a time.

If you did make it all the way through, don't let this be a standing point or a plateau – let this be your beginning, the kickstart you need to ensure that you stay this way – happy, healthy and the best version of you that you can be. And not just for you, but for the people who look up to you.

Your body will be in fat-burning mode now, so you need to take care of it and fuel the fire. Keep going with the clean, lean foods. Don't fall back into cake and cookies every day. You don't need to eat sugar. A punnet of raspberries or blueberries will satisfy a sweet craving. And then look forward to a little treat on the weekend, not a feast.

Remember that you need water – lots of it! Water is key to keeping your body functioning the way you want it to. You literally cannot function without it, and you absolutely can't burn fat. Your water intake should remain at a minimum of 2 litres (70 fl oz/8 cups) per day, or 3 litres (105 fl oz/12 cups) if you can manage it. Drinking that amount of water and getting the right amount of sleep could be the two best habits you will ever form.

Above all, don't lose your motivation to get to training or to sweat a little. Exercise is a reward for a healthy life, not a punishment for a bad diet. You have come so far in the last 8 weeks and I know you can keep it up. You have what it takes, you honestly do. You need to keep that incredible fitness you have worked so hard for. It's so hard to get it, but so easy to lose. Maintenance of your fitness is also vital to keeping your heart happy.

There's nothing wrong with having a treat – you worked hard for it! And what is life if it isn't made up of our favourite foods, shared culinary experiences, and enjoying tastes from restaurants and childhood memories? But just remember, if you have two, three or four days of eating the old stuff you used to eat and drinking in excess, you will be chasing your tail for weeks – mentally and physically. If you value the health that you have given yourself over the last 8 weeks, be kind to yourself. Create some new recipes, or go for a healthier version of what you would usually have.

Whenever I look at something I really want to eat, I ask myself, 'Will this be the last time I'll have an opportunity to eat this particular food?' It's very unlikely that it is, so think about it. Just having a few mouthfuls that you really savour and enjoy is much better for you than devouring a huge portion and regretting it.

In short:

+ Eat unhealthy and you will look unhealthy.
+ If you don't drink enough water, your body won't recover as fast and your metabolism will slow down.
+ Put in 50% at training and you'll get 50% back. Do you only want to be okay-ish? Or do you want to look and feel 100% amazing?

+ If you eat healthy during the week and feast on the weekend, you'll constantly be trying to catch up.
+ If you want to achieve something, then you have to put in the effort. Maintaining where you want to be is definitely easier than getting there in the first place, so don't let yourself slide. Feed the engine: keep moving the goal posts and achieving new goals.

You are strong! Don't ever let that thought waver. If you think back to 8 weeks ago, you'll realise how far you've come. So don't stop now – push through and start working towards your next goals.

Take some 'after' photos and sit them beside your 'before' photos. And then give yourself a high-five, a pat on the back and a huge smile, because YOU DID IT. And with that success comes much more. You can achieve anything – this is just the start of the new you. All you have to do is work for it.

STAY STRONG

`Em & Chief`

INDEX

2015 Hella yeah salad 190

alcohol 24–5
Anastasi, Andy 82–3
anchovies: 2015 Hella yeah salad 190
Asian-style mussels 154
asparagus
    Asparagus, bacon and ricotta frittatas 198
    Cauliflower fried rice 208
    Cream of asparagus soup 146
    Parmesan poached eggs with asparagus 171
    Prosciutto-wrapped asparagus 142
Asparagus, bacon and ricotta frittatas 198
Avo smash 160
avocados
    Avo smash 160
    Bacon and avocado fries 211
    BEATS (bacon, egg, avocado and tomato salad) 165
    Crab and avocado rolls 138
    Smashed avocado and feta on protein bread 181
    Taco-less tacos 210

bacon
    Asparagus, bacon and ricotta frittatas 198
    Bacon and avocado fries 211
    Bacon and egg cups 189
    BEATS (bacon, egg, avocado and tomato salad) 165
    Breakfast bacon bruschetta 135
    Brussels sprouts and bacon hash 172
    BZB fritters 160
    Carbonara 150
    Cauliflower fried rice 208
Bacon and avocado fries 211
Bacon and egg cups 189
Baked salmon with mushies and spinach 142
Barbecued chicken tikka kebabs 202
Barbecued chilli octopus with garlic yoghurt 151
Barbecued salmon 147
barramundi: Oven-cooked barramundi 150
basil
    BZB fritters 160
    Combination rissoles 152

    Mediterranean baked fish 141
bean sprouts: Easy chicken stir-fry 176
Beasley, Dustin 120–1
BEATS (bacon, egg, avocado and tomato salad) 165
beef
    Beef schnitzel with mushroom sauce 204
    Caribbean beef 173
    Devil nachos 183
    Eggplant lasagne 162
    Grilled beef, sweet potato and rocket salad 212
    Hot and sour beef soup with lime 148
    Mexican stuffed capsicums 166
    Sweet onion meatballs 200
    Taco-less tacos 210
Beef schnitzel with mushroom sauce 204
breadcrumbs: Stuffed mushrooms 168
breads 28, 78
Breakfast bacon bruschetta 135
Breakfast casserole to go 145
broccoli: Chicken and vegetable casserole 184
brussels sprouts
    Brussels sprouts and bacon hash 172
    Italian chicken with brussels sprouts 168
Brussels sprouts and bacon hash 172
burritos: Inferno burrito 154
Butterfly chicken with rosemary 198
BZB fritters 160

cabbage
    Cauliflower fried rice 208
    Chicken and vegetable casserole 184
capsicums
    2015 Hella yeah salad 190
    Breakfast casserole to go 145
    Cauliflower fried rice 208
    Chicken and vegetable casserole 184
    Chicken curry in a hurry 178
    Easy chicken stir-fry 176
    Huevos a la ranchera 189
    Mexican stuffed capsicums 166
    Pork larb in lettuce cups 138
    Taco-less tacos 210

Zucchini gazpacho with diced red capsicum 146
Carbonara 150
Caribbean beef 173
carrots
    Cauliflower fried rice 208
    Taco-less tacos 210
case studies
    Anastasi, Andy 82–3
    Beasley, Dustin 120–1
    Dooley, Patrick 106–7
    Giaquinto, Connie 114–15
    Hames, Rosie Alys 128–9
    Ratnasinghe, Christina 70–1
    Rea, Charleen 98–9
    Sebastian, Guy 16–17
    Sebastian, Jules 18–19
    Wokes, Rebecca 90–1
    Wokes, Richard 90–1
cauliflower
    Cauliflower fried rice 208
    Cauliflower rissoles 172
Cauliflower fried rice 208
Cauliflower rissoles 172
cheddar cheese
    Eggplant lasagne 162
    Skillet breakfast 171
cheese see cheddar cheese; cottage cheese; cream cheese; feta;
mozzarella; parmesan; ricotta
chicken
    Barbecued chicken tikka kebabs 202
    Butterfly chicken with rosemary 198
    Carbonara 150
    Chicken and vegetable casserole 184
    Chicken curry in a hurry 178
    Combination rissoles 152
    Easy chicken stir-fry 176
    Greek chicken salad with tzatziki 140
    Inferno burrito 154
    Italian chicken with brussels sprouts 168
    Super-easy peri-peri chicken 193
    Sweet onion meatballs 200
    Taco-less tacos 210
    Thai green curry chicken balls 194
Chicken and vegetable casserole 184
Chicken curry in a hurry 178
chillies: Barbecued chilli octopus with garlic yoghurt 151
chocolate: Mocha shake 156
coffee: Mocha shake 156
Combination rissoles 152

coriander
    Chicken curry in a hurry 178
    Hot and sour beef soup with lime 148
    Thai green curry chicken balls 194
cottage cheese
    Cottage cheese and devilled eggs 186
    Oven-cooked barramundi 150
Cottage cheese and devilled eggs 186
Crab and avocado rolls 138
cream
    Eggplant lasagne 162
    Pork and fennel patties 197
cream cheese
    2015 Hella yeah salad 190
    Chicken and vegetable casserole 184
    Crab and avocado rolls 138
    Mint curry omelette 207
Cream of asparagus soup 146
Cucumber refresher 169
cucumbers
    Crab and avocado rolls 138
    Cucumber refresher 169
    Greek chicken salad with tzatziki 140
    Pulled pork salad 186
    Super-easy peri-peri chicken 193
    Taco-less tacos 210
curries
    Chicken curry in a hurry 178
    Grilled curried fish 203
    Thai green curry chicken balls 194

dairy foods 27, 78
DARC Protocol 32–65
Devil nachos 183
Dooley, Patrick 106–7
dressings: Ranch dressing 165
drinks 29, 79

Easy chicken stir-fry 176
Eggplant lasagne 162
eggplants
    Eggplant lasagne 162
    Foil-roasted eggplant 174
    Moussaka 164
eggs 27, 78
    Bacon and egg cups 189
    BEATS (bacon, egg, avocado and tomato salad) 165
    Beef schnitzel with mushroom sauce 204
    Breakfast casserole to go 145

Brussels sprouts and bacon hash 172
BZB fritters 160
Carbonara 150
Cauliflower fried rice 208
Cottage cheese and devilled eggs 186
Devil nachos 183
Huevos a la ranchera 189
Inferno burrito 154
Mexican breakfast 159
Mint curry omelette 207
Moussaka 164
Parmesan poached eggs with asparagus 171
Pommy Scotch eggs 211
Protein pancakes 136
Sausage rolls 201
Skillet breakfast 171

fennel: Pork and fennel patties 197
feta
    2015 Hella yeah salad 190
    Bacon and egg cups 189
    Moussaka 164
    Pulled pork salad 186
    Sautéed spinach 192
    Smashed avocado and feta on protein bread 181
fettuccine: Carbonara 150
fish
    Baked salmon with mushies and spinach 142
    Barbecued salmon 147
    Fish with herbs 152
    Fishy rissoles 193
    Grilled curried fish 203
    Mediterranean baked fish 141
    Oven-cooked barramundi 150
    Thyme salmon fillets 192
    see also seafood
Fish with herbs 152
Fishy rissoles 193
Foil-roasted eggplant 174
frittatas
    Asparagus, bacon and ricotta frittata 198
    Zucchini and ricotta frittata 182
fritters: BZB fritters 160
fruit 28, 102, 110

garlic
    2015 Hella yeah salad 190
    Barbecued chilli octopus with garlic yoghurt 151
    Zesty lemon grilled calamari with garlic 174

Giaquinto, Connie 114–15
grains 28, 78, 102, 124
Greek chicken salad with tzatziki 140
Green tea frozen yoghurt 169
greens 26, 75, 76
Grilled beef, sweet potato and rocket salad 212
Grilled curried fish 203
Grilled scallops wrapped in ham 176

ham: Grilled scallops wrapped in ham 176
Hames, Rosie Alys 128–9
herbs 29, 79
    Fish with herbs 152
Hot and sour beef soup with lime 148
Huevos a la ranchera 189

ice cream: Protein ice cream 156
Inferno burrito 154
Italian chicken with brussels sprouts 168

lamb
    Moussaka 164
    Sweet onion meatballs 200
lasagne: Eggplant lasagne 162
lemons: Zesty lemon grilled calamari with garlic 174
lettuce
    2015 Hella yeah salad 190
    Oven-cooked barramundi 150
    Pork larb in lettuce cups 138
limes
    Cucumber refresher 169
    Hot and sour beef soup with lime 148

meatballs: Sweet onion meatballs 200
meats 27, 78
Mediterranean baked fish 141
Mexican breakfast 159
Mexican stuffed capsicums 166
milk: Mocha shake 156
mint
    Greek chicken salad with tzatziki 140
    Mint curry omelette 207
Mint curry omelette 207
Mocha shake 156
Moussaka 164
mozzarella: Pork and fennel patties 197
mushrooms
    2015 Hella yeah salad 190
    Baked salmon with mushies and spinach 142

Beef schnitzel with mushroom sauce 204
Brussels sprouts and bacon hash 172
Cauliflower fried rice 208
Mexican stuffed capsicums 166
Skillet breakfast 171
Stuffed mushrooms 168
Taco-less tacos 210
mussels: Asian-style mussels 154

nachos: Devil nachos 183
noodles 28, 78
nuts 94

octopus: Barbecued chilli octopus with garlic yoghurt 151
oils 94
omelettes: Mint curry omelette 207
onions: Sweet onion meatballs 200
Oven-cooked barramundi 150

pancakes: Protein pancakes 136
parmesan
    Breakfast bacon bruschetta 135
    Carbonara 150
    Cauliflower rissoles 172
    Chicken and vegetable casserole 184
    Eggplant lasagne 162
    Parmesan poached eggs with asparagus 171
    Stuffed mushrooms 168
Parmesan poached eggs with asparagus 171
pasta: Carbonara 150
patties: Pork and fennel patties 197
peri-peri: Super-easy peri-peri chicken 193
Pommy Scotch eggs 211
pork
    Breakfast casserole to go 145
    Combination rissoles 152
    Pork and fennel patties 197
    Pork larb in lettuce cups 138
    Pulled pork salad 186
    Sausage rolls 201
    Sweet onion meatballs 200
    Taco-less tacos 210
Pork and fennel patties 197
Pork larb in lettuce cups 138
portion control 122–3
prawns: Combination rissoles 152
Prosciutto-wrapped asparagus 142
protein bars 116–17
protein bread

Devil nachos 183
Sausage rolls 201
Smashed avocado and feta on protein bread 181
Stuffed mushrooms 168
Protein Bread Co. 123
Protein ice cream 156
Protein pancakes 136
protein powder 117
    Protein ice cream 156
    Protein pancakes 136
Pulled pork salad 186

Ranch dressing 165
Ratnasinghe, Christina 70–1
Rea, Sharleen 98–9
restricted foods 27
ricotta
    Asparagus, bacon and ricotta frittatas 198
    Mint curry omelette 207
    Protein ice cream 156
    Zucchini and ricotta frittata 182
rissoles
    Cauliflower rissoles 172
    Combination rissoles 152
    Fishy rissoles 193
rocket: Grilled beef, sweet potato and rocket salad 212
rosemary: Butterfly chicken with rosemary 198

salads
    2015 Hella yeah salad 190
    BEATS (bacon, egg, avocado and tomato salad) 165
    Greek chicken salad with tzatziki 140
    Grilled beef, sweet potato and rocket salad 212
    Pulled pork salad 186
salmon
    Baked salmon with mushies and spinach 142
    Barbecued salmon 147
    Thyme salmon fillets 192
Sausage rolls 201
Sautéed spinach 192
scallops: Grilled scallops wrapped in ham 176
seafood 27, 78
    Asian-style mussels 154
    Barbecued chilli octopus with garlic yoghurt 151
    Combination rissoles 152
    Grilled scallops wrapped in ham 176
    Zesty lemon grilled calamari with garlic 174
    see also fish
Sebastian, Guy 16–17

Sebastian, Jules 18–19
Skillet breakfast 171
sleep 86–7
Smashed avocado and feta on protein bread 181
soups
    Cream of asparagus soup 146
    Hot and sour beef soup with lime 148
    Zucchini gazpacho with diced red capsicum 146
spices 29, 79
spinach
    Baked salmon with mushies and spinach 142
    Breakfast bacon bruschetta 135
    Mediterranean baked fish 141
    Pulled pork salad 186
    Sautéed spinach 192
    Skillet breakfast 171
    Super-easy peri-peri chicken 193
    Thai green curry chicken balls 194
spring onions: Chicken curry in a hurry 178
squid: Zesty lemon grilled calamari with garlic 174
Stuffed mushrooms 168
sugar 116–17
Super-easy peri-peri chicken 193
Sweet onion meatballs 200
sweet potato: Grilled beef, sweet potato and rocket salad 212

Taco-less tacos 210
Thai green curry chicken balls 194
Thyme salmon fillets 192
tomatoes
    Baked salmon with mushies and spinach 142
    BEATS (bacon, egg, avocado and tomato salad) 165
    Devil nachos 183
    Eggplant lasagne 162
    Greek chicken salad with tzatziki 140
    Huevos a la ranchera 189
    Italian chicken with brussels sprouts 168
    Mediterranean baked fish 141
    Mexican breakfast 159
    Moussaka 164
    Pulled pork salad 186
    Taco-less tacos 210
turkey: Pommy Scotch eggs 211
tzatziki: Greek chicken salad with tzatziki 140

vegetables 26, 76, 94
    Chicken and vegetable casserole 184

water 24, 75
weight loss, versus fat loss 101
Wokes, Rebecca 90–1
Wokes, Richard 90–1

yoghurt
    Barbecued chicken tikka kebabs 202
    Barbecued chilli octopus with garlic yoghurt 151
    Greek chicken salad with tzatziki 140
    Green tea frozen yoghurt 169
    Mexican stuffed capsicums 166
    Moussaka 164
    Protein ice cream 156
    Protein pancakes 136
    Ranch dressing 165

Zesty lemon grilled calamari with garlic 174
zucchini
    BZB fritters 160
    Cauliflower fried rice 208
    Chicken and vegetable casserole 184
    Combination rissoles 152
    Grilled beef, sweet potato and rocket salad 212
    Zucchini and ricotta frittata 182
    Zucchini gazpacho with diced red capsicum 146
Zucchini and ricotta frittata 182
Zucchini gazpacho with diced red capsicum 146

THANKS, TRIBE!

Writing a book is a daunting and exciting experience, and over the last decade of running the 8 Weeks to Wow program, we have had the pleasure of welcoming so many people, from all around the world to our ever-growing tribe of success stories.

Thank you so much for trusting in our methods and becoming a part of our team. Without **YOU**, there would be no library of new and exciting recipes, no helpful suggestions and no feedback as to how we can make sure you are all excelling and making the most of the 8 weeks you have put aside for this. Big, big thanks to these guys from our 8WTW community for their recipe contributions, which appear in this book: Harry, Sharkey and Dani, Connie, Rosie, Rochelle (Pixie!), Ernie, Matt, Bron, Jo, Kylie, Gerry, Rita, Em, Crystal, Erin, Angela and Larissa. You guys are legends!

A special thanks to publisher Kelly Doust for seeing something in our program that she could translate into everybody's language and for helping us and encouraging us to stay true to our authentic and true selves. She saw the whole package and was with us every step of the way.

Thank you so much to Katie Bosher, the team at Northwood Green and to editor Justine Harding for being so supportive and understanding of our deadlines and being just the right amount of 'get it done' and 'let's try this'.

Thank you to Jeremy Simons, our amazing photographer for capturing the true essence of us as coaches (and making us look badass). Your ideas and imagery were beyond incredible. Thanks as well to Elsa Morgan for hair and makeup, and to Justine Poole and Grace Campbell for such a beautiful and fun food shoot. Big thanks goes to photographer Ondrej Garaj for the great step-by-step workout shots, and of course to our amazing fitness models Patrick (Dools) and Maria.

And last, but most certainly not least, thanks to the eleven members of our 8WTW tribe who shared their transformation stories for this book. Putting yourself in print for the world to see is so brave, and you are our heroes – you look like superheroes!

THANK YOU!

Published in 2018 by Murdoch Books, an imprint of Allen & Unwin

Murdoch Books Australia
83 Alexander Street
Crows Nest NSW 2065
Phone: +61 (0)2 8425 0100
murdochbooks.com.au
info@murdochbooks.com.au

Murdoch Books UK
Ormond House
26–27 Boswell Street
London WC1N 3JZ
Phone: +44 (0) 20 8785 5995
murdochbooks.co.uk
info@murdochbooks.co.uk

For Corporate Orders & Custom Publishing, contact our Business
Development Team at
salesenquiries@murdochbooks.com.au.

Publisher: Kelly Doust
Editorial Manager: Katie Bosher
Creative Direction: northwoodgreen.com
Project Editor: Justine Harding
Photographer: Jeremy Simons
Stylist: Justine Poole
Home Economist: Grace Campbell
Hair and Make-up: Elsa Morgan
Production Director: Lou Playfair

Text © Emilie Brabon-Hames and James 'Chief' Brabon 2018
The moral right of the authors has been asserted.
Design © Murdoch Books 2018

Photography © Jeremy Simons 2018 except for the following:
Step-by-step exercise images pages 43–65 © Ondrej Garaj 2018;
'Before' photo page 17 and back cover by Jason Lee; 'After' photos
pages 17, 19 and back cover, and 'Before' photo on page 19 by Jason
Ierace; 'After' photos pages 71, 107, 115 and 129 by Benito Martin;
'After' photo page 99 by Andy McColl.
Cover photography by Jeremy Simons

Magazine covers on page 4 appear courtesy of Pacific Magazines.

Every reasonable effort has been made to trace the owners of
copyright materials in this book, but in some instances this has
proven impossible. The author(s) and publisher will be glad to
receive information leading to more complete acknowledgements
in subsequent printings of the book and in the meantime extend
their apologies for any omissions.

All rights reserved. No part of this publication may be reproduced,
stored in a retrieval system or transmitted in any form or by
any means, electronic, mechanical, photocopying, recording or
otherwise, without the prior written permission of the publisher.

A cataloguing-in-publication entry is available from the catalogue
of the National Library of Australia at nla.gov.au.

ISBN 978 1 7605 237 32 Australia
ISBN 978 1 7606 346 67 UK

A catalogue record for this book is available from the British Library.

Colour reproduction by Splitting Image Colour Studio Pty Ltd,
Clayton, Victoria
Printed by Hang Tai Printing Company Limited, China

IMPORTANT: Those who might be at risk from the effects of salmonella poisoning (the elderly, pregnant women, young children and those suffering from immune deficiency diseases) should consult their doctor with any concerns about eating raw eggs.

DISCLAIMER: The information and suggestions in this book are for your consideration only and may not be suitable to your particular circumstances. We are not recommending that people eat certain foods or follow any particular dietary advice. This is particularly so if you have allergies or other conditions that may give rise to adverse reactions to certain foods or diets. Before undertaking any of the suggestions in this book, therefore, we strongly recommend that you consult your own healthcare professional. Neither the authors nor the publisher accepts any liability or responsibility for any loss or damage suffered or incurred as a result of undertaking or following any suggestions contained in this book.

OVEN GUIDE: You may find cooking times vary depending on the oven you are using. For fan-forced ovens, as a general rule, set the oven temperature to 20°C (70°F) lower than indicated in the recipe.
MEASURES GUIDE: We have used 20 ml (4 teaspoon) tablespoon measures. If you are using a 15 ml (3 teaspoon) tablespoon add an extra teaspoon of the ingredient for each tablespoon specified.